JOHN VIDAL (1949–2023) was born and brought up in West Africa. One of the world's most experienced environment journalists, he worked for over thirty years on the frontlines of the global war against nature. As environment editor of the *Guardian*, he reported on the climate crisis, disease and ecological change from more than 100 countries, during which time he was attacked by loggers and farmers, imprisoned by whalers and sued by oil and chemical companies. Vidal won many national and international awards for his writing and film-making. He was the author of one previous book and contributed chapters to books on war, famine and conservation.

FEVERED PLANET

How Diseases Emerge When We Harm Nature

JOHN VIDAL

BLOOMSBURY PUBLISHING

LONDON · OXFORD · NEW YORK · NEW DELHI · SYDNEY

BLOOMSBURY PUBLISHING
Bloomsbury Publishing Plc
50 Bedford Square, London, WC1B 3DP, UK
29 Earlsfort Terrace, Dublin 2, Ireland

BLOOMSBURY, BLOOMSBURY PUBLISHING and the Diana logo are trademarks of
Bloomsbury Publishing Plc

First published in Great Britain, 2023
This edition published 2024

A catalogue record for this book is available from the British Library

ISBN: HB: 978-1-5266-3227-2; TPB: 978-1-5266-3228-9; PB: 978-1-5266-3229-6;
EBOOK: 978-1-5266-3219-7; EPDF: 978-1-5266-6669-7

2 4 6 8 10 9 7 5 3 1

Typeset by Newgen KnowledgeWorks Pvt. Ltd., Chennai, India
Printed and bound in Great Britain by CPI Group (UK) Ltd, Croydon CR0 4YY

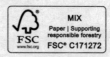

To find out more about our authors and books visit www.bloomsbury.com
and sign up for our newsletters

CONTENTS

INTRODUCTION: TIP OF THE ICEBERG

If the misery of the poor be caused not by the laws of nature,
but by our institutions, great is our sin.

Charles Darwin, *Voyage of the Beagle*, 1839

It seemed an endless journey by plane, boat, bus and motorbike
to reach Mayibout 2, a small village close to the unmarked Gabon
border with Congo and Cameroon. I had come to within a few
kilometres of the equator line to understand how a deadly viral
disease called Ebola had spilled out of the great Minkébé jungle in
a series of small epidemics in 1994.

Mayibout 2 was the site of only the fourth known outbreak
of Ebola, one of the deadliest viruses ever recorded. Over several
months it had invaded half a dozen Gabonese villages close to the
forest. Medical researchers thought that it had jumped first from
a host animal like a bat or a rat into a chimp or a monkey, whose
infected blood or meat had then been consumed by humans. But
mystery and terror still surrounded the disease, and everyone was
shocked at the way the virus caused the human body to bleed
profusely from every orifice before it quickly killed.

The last fifty kilometres had been along deeply rutted tracks
which branched off into many smaller paths constructed by
loggers to get their machinery deeper into the forest; several small,
makeshift artisanal gold mines were operating and polluting rivers.
We passed logging camps in forest clearings with piles of precious
afrormosia logs waiting to be shipped to Europe or China, as well

as groups of indigenous Baka people, and hunters in ragged clothes carrying traps and small antelopes over their shoulders.

We reached Mayibout 2 in the afternoon rain, drenched and exhausted, to be met by Bob Lucien, the chief, who appeared still broken by the disease that had devastated his village six years earlier before seemingly disappearing back into the forest. We walked slowly past simple graves and through clusters of small huts. The community of about sixty families was spread along 400 metres of the great Ivindo river, a tributary of a tributary of the mighty Congo. On the far bank the forest was a great green wall, the domain of gorillas, monkeys and forest elephants.

We shared a warm Regab beer at a rudimentary riverside bar and Lucien recounted how Ebola had come to Mayibout. A group of village youths, hunting with a dog in the forest, had found a dead chimpanzee and carried it back for people to cook and share. That was not unusual, he said, and it was quite acceptable and welcome to eat 'bush', or wild, meat like this. The illness that soon engulfed those who had shared the meal was first assumed to be malaria, a common enough problem in Mayibout, but shortly it became clear that this was far more serious. 'What started with a headache soon became a high fever, then people lost consciousness,' he said.

Like so many communities throughout history when confronted by plague or a pandemic, Mayibout had panicked, he said. Those who could took to boats or ran away, others locked down, and neighbouring villages stayed clear. The ministry of health was told, and white men in hazmat suits from the globally funded International Centre for Medical Research in Franceville (CIRMF), 150 kilometres away, arrived to confirm that the mystery disease was the dreaded Ebola. The village, already isolated by its geography, was shut down. 'That's when we knew we would die,' said Lucien.

By then it was too late. Within days, twenty-one people who had butchered, eaten or just touched the blood of the chimp had died and others hung between life and death. Lucien, terrified, shut himself and his family in his hut for a week, not daring to go out and nearly starving. His friend Nesto, who contracted the disease, was taken with others by canoe down the river to the regional capital town of Makouko, where he recovered after three weeks in hospital. 'Many, many people died. Some who left never returned,' he said.

By now other villagers had gathered around us at the bar. I asked them why they thought Ebola had come to Mayibout. It was a 'malediction' and 'sorcery', not caused by humans but the divine, they said. I asked them whether they had seen major changes in the nearby forest in the years before the disease had come, and they all mentioned logging and mining. But could logging or mining have led to the emergence of Ebola, I asked. No, they insisted. That was 'development', which brought jobs and money.

I spent the day in the village hearing stories of how the village had been cursed, and how people still feared to go into the forest to hunt. For a more scientific view I travelled on to the CIRMF in Franceville. The equivalent of Porton Down in the UK, or Fort Detrick in the US, this was Africa's most important great apes research centre, with its own chimp colony. It also had one of the continent's only two high-security biological laboratories where work on Ebola, HIV/Aids, malaria, Marburg, coronaviruses and other deadly pathogens was done. It was from here that virologists had sped to Mayibout 2 and other Congo-basin Ebola outbreaks when it first emerged in southern Sudan. The site was heavily guarded by high fences and men with guns. Only a handful of people were allowed to enter some of the buildings.

Eric Leroy, the chief virologist there, had spent several years trying to find the reservoir host of the Ebola virus, travelling to the outbreaks. He suspected the host animal was a bat but was not yet certain. He looked like a classic old-school French colonial administrator in his suit and tie, but was in fact a highly driven disease-outbreak veterinarian, well used to life in the Congolese forests. He and his team of virus hunters had just returned from weeks collecting and analysing samples of saliva, faeces and blood from bats and animals that they or bushmeat hunters had trapped. It was gruelling, dangerous frontline research and many new discoveries had been made. After collecting genetic material close to places where people or animals were known to have been infected with Ebola, his team were increasingly convinced that fruit bats were the prime reservoir of disease. Later analysis would prove him to be correct.

We discussed Ebola's possible origins and as I was leaving I asked Leroy if he or his team could see any link between the emergence of Ebola in Gabon and the global loss of forests or climate change, or even the growth in human numbers. They were unfair questions that I don't think he or many other scientists had much considered or had time for. He paused before answering. 'Possibly. Possibly.' I left, hearing the cries of what were probably the chimps in one of the heavily guarded, fortress-like buildings of the maximum security establishment which I had not been allowed to enter.

* * *

I returned to London in turmoil. Until I went to Mayibout it had barely occurred to me that human diseases could be linked to the planetary-scale changes we were seeing in the environment, like deforestation, warming temperatures or the loss of habitat. But Ebola had made me think about the underlying causes of disease, how vulnerable we all may be and how responsible we in the rich North might be for what happens half a world away.

Like most people in wealthy countries, I had little first-hand experience of disease, let alone a pandemic that no one had had any defence against. Despite being born in Africa and travelling frequently throughout the tropics, I had always felt well protected by vaccines and pills. Disease happened to others, I had always assumed, and the idea that in this day of advanced medicine a minute pathogen could invade a community without warning or precedent and kill nearly everyone it touched was shocking. I shuddered to think what might happen if Ebola or some other fatal new viral disease that could kill so many people so fast ever spread in a wealthy country. Like the people of Mayibout I had no concept that nature could be so brutal, and little idea that the environment we all depend on for food and well-being could so monstrously turn against us.

I had been covering what was broadly termed 'environment' for the *Guardian* since 1989. It was a fast-growing, alarming roller-coaster of a journalistic brief and one that was both depressing and thrilling. Bird, mammal and amphibian numbers were in freefall; pollution from fossil fuels was poisoning the air and land and killing millions of people every year. Climate change was now kicking in and threatening existential change, and every year brought evidence of more plant and tree diseases, as well as extreme droughts and floods. The world was physically changing before our eyes and on a planetary level, the collapse of nature seemed far more dramatic and newsworthy than anything happening in London, Washington or Sydney. Telling the stories of the extraordinary, inspiring people I was meeting on every continent who were protesting at what was happening and trying to protect the natural world was the reward for the depressing litany of natural loss and decline.

I was no scientist but it was not hard to see why it was happening. Simultaneously with the collapse of nature, the last thirty years had also seen a great surge in human activity. It could be seen in the speed at which people moved, the longer distances they travelled, the fast-growing populations and the swelling cities. The sheer number of people and domestic animals, the amount of food being grown and eaten, the minerals being mined, the forests being felled and the goods being made and consumed were all heavily impacting the planet.

And the more I looked the more it made sense that there were strong links between disease and the environment. There was indeed a precedent for Ebola. Mayibout 2 was just 150 or so kilometres from the Sangha river in southern Cameroon, where another deadly viral disease called HIV/Aids had almost certainly been circulating since the 1920s, at first among chimpanzees before it crossed to humans and became a pandemic around 1981. Somehow – a local hunter butchering monkey meat, hungry soldiers at the end of the First World War, even a European vaccine trial gone wrong – the HIV virus had jumped into humans and been transported down trade routes and rivers to the great Congolese capital city of Kinshasa. From there it spread rapidly via international workers and travellers, eventually reaching the gay community in the US and the rest of the world. In just forty years it had become the deadliest pandemic known to humans since the 1919–20 influenza from which up to 50 million people had died, and there was still no vaccine.

Was it a coincidence that two of the world's most deadly diseases had emerged so close to each other and within a few years, in areas where previously untouched rainforest was being devastated by road building, logging, mining and people moving in? It seemed highly unlikely. Both pandemics had been blamed on poor people eating animals, but this seemed too convenient an explanation. I checked the World Health Organization's situation reports for all known Ebola outbreaks and, sure enough, most mentioned in the small print that the disease had emerged, just as in Mayibout, close to areas of deforestation and human destruction of the jungle. Similar to HIV/Aids, the disease may have been started by hunters but their entry to the forests was facilitated by loggers' roads. Was that significant? I did not know, but I began to wonder.

I talked to epidemiologists and vets at the World Health Organization in Geneva and the World Organisation for Animal Health in Paris, the two global bodies charged with monitoring human and animal diseases. Both were beginning to make links between disease and ecological disturbance, but there was little research being done. What was certain was that new infectious diseases, especially those linked to animals, were emerging throughout the world.

* * *

Twenty years on, in the midst of the Covid-19 pandemic that by January 2023 had already killed 6.7 million people, infected over 650 million and cost trillions of dollars to contain, we can look back and understand that HIV/Aids and Ebola were just warning shots in humanity's long war against infectious diseases. In quick succession since the 1990s, at least thirty dangerous new diseases, none of which were predicted or prepared for, have emerged in different parts of the world. Some, like SARS and bird flu, have killed thousands of people and created global panic; many, such as Marburg, Lassa fever, Mpox, MERS, Hendra and Nipah, have been more or less contained, by good fortune as much as by good science. Others, like tuberculosis, cholera and dengue, which plagued the ancient world, have re-emerged with new vigour, and yet more, like West Nile virus and Zika, have mutated into more serious diseases and jumped continents. But while there are vaccines and cures for some of these diseases, none has been eradicated, and it is likely that there are more infectious diseases in the world today than at any other time in history, as well as more outbreaks in more countries.

The urgent question now is whether harming the planet also harms human health and, if so, what links these new diseases, why are they emerging now and what is driving them? My instinct twenty years ago was that their roots lay in the damage humans were causing to the planet by the way we farm, live and eat, but was I wrong? What is the evidence? Are we really changing the balance between the natural world and humans, exploiting the world's resources and creating the perfect conditions for diseases like Covid-19 to emerge and spread far and wide? I wanted to find out.

This book is the result of a journalistic exploration conducted in many countries over the last twenty years to see how far the growing number of human, plant and animal diseases that we face today is linked to the worsening human-made ecological crises of which the loss of the natural world and climate change are just two. I wanted to see what evidence there was and draw together the many strands linking disease and the planetary environment.

The first part traces the roots of human disease from the birth of animal farming and the emergence of cities to the European colonisation of other continents and the industrial revolution; the second part investigates how the many diseases now emerging are being driven by human action and reflect the degradation of the planet; and the third part shows how a great pandemic like Covid-19 may be just the tip of an iceberg of more deadly and disruptive diseases to come if we do not change course. Finally, it is a story of hope, showing that it is entirely possible to reverse a great deal of the damage done and both heal the planet and keep ourselves free of disease.

The journey to join the dots between our health and that of the planet, and understand how humanity's disruption of the environment may have led to deadly diseases through the ages, starts with a mound of rubble in what is today one of the most desolate and unforgiving places on earth – but which only 13,000 years ago was a land of milk and honey, and of people in remarkably good health.

Pathogens, politics and scientific theory all evolve rapidly, so it's natural that some statistics or situations discussed in this book will have changed between the short time it goes to press and when it is published. For instance, as I write in April 2023, arguments over the origins of Covid-19 are still not resolved, avian flu is moving relentlessly from birds to mammals and many diseases with pandemic potential are emerging and spreading to new places. Only time will tell if they will change the world.

PART I

CHANGING LANDSCAPES

The will to live exists in every being, even in the tiniest; it is present as completely as in all that ever were, are and will be, taken together.

Arthur Schopenhauer, *Parego and Paralipomena*, 1851

1

STIRRING THE MICROBIAL POT ...

It is May 2014. Turkey has diverted the headwaters of the mighty river Euphrates, causing the level of Lake Assad 800 kilometres to the south in northern Syria to drop six metres in a few months. It is the start of a long battle by three armies to control the Tabqa Dam, the largest in the Middle East.

In the hands first of the Syrian government, then of the opposition forces and from 2016 of the Islamic State army, the great earth and concrete barrier at the southern end of the huge reservoir controls the electricity and irrigation of the whole region. Battles raged for three years until the dam was eventually captured in 2017 by Syrian troops backed by 200 American special forces in one of the most decisive confrontations of the war.

All three armies threatened to blow up the dam and if any one of them had succeeded, or if Turkey to the north had allowed the water levels to carry on falling, a great mound of earth, rock and debris about 500 metres long and eight metres high would have been exposed on a small raised plateau. It is all that remains of the ruined Neolithic settlement of Abu Hureyra, which had been flooded when the reservoir was filled in 1971.

That drowned mound of rubble marks a critical point in humanity's evolution and the origin of infectious and animal-borne, or zoonotic, diseases. It was here, or somewhere like here, around 13,000 years ago that the Neolithic revolution got under way when people started to settle down and domesticate animals like the pig, the sheep and the goat. It was from places like this that many of the ancestors of modern diseases like the common cold, influenza, cholera, smallpox, even an early form of SARS or coronavirus, would have emerged and spread around the world.[1]

Abu Hureyra was evacuated just before the Tabqa Dam was filled with water in 1971. What archaeologists Andrew Moore from University College London and others found when sifting through the debris of nearly 10,000 years of continuous occupation was not one but two settlements. One was an ancient Natufian village of semi-nomadic hunter-gatherers dating to around 13,500 BC; the other was a village of sedentary farmers, 4,000 years younger, whose inhabitants grew crops and reared animals for food.

The land around Abu Hureyra is now war-torn, drought-prone and suffers permanent water shortages, a far cry from the mild climate, abundance and diversity that would have existed at the time of the settlements that Moore and his colleagues discovered. Abu Hureyra lies on what would have been the banks of the Euphrates in the heart of the Fertile Crescent – that great arc of lands stretching from the Nile and northern Egypt through Jordan, Palestine and Syria to Iraq and Iran – which 13,000 years ago enjoyed some of the most attractive conditions of life imaginable. The climate was warm, the sun shone and there was plenty of fertile land and fresh water, as well as deep rich soil and shaded valleys filled with grasses and wild animals to hunt.

In his great book *After the Ice*, Steven Mithen, professor of archaeology at Reading University, paints a thrilling picture of the good life there. 'Here on the banks of the river daily life at Hureyra begins. The gazelle do not appear and the hunters leave to search the river valley for wild pigs and asses. The women and children work in the gardens, weeding, killing bugs and collecting whatever has ripened in the sun and reap a rich harvest.'[2]

To get some idea of the richness of the diet and the abundance of food eaten, a modern healthy diet may include about ten plants and fruits. But in the first, older Abu Hureyra village the archaeologists found evidence that 192 species of plants were eaten, including rye, lentils and wheat. The animals eaten were all wild.

Yet in the younger, larger village, people had changed lifestyles and diets, switching from hunting and gathering food to herding domesticated animals and growing crops. Instead of eating hundreds of plants and seeds collected from close by, they now grew just a few grain crops, many originating far away.

Seeds collected there show they grew emmer and einkorn, single-grain wheats from what is now Palestine and northern Syria, as well as chickpeas from Turkey. Sheep and goats, and later cattle and pigs, were kept and eaten, and the soil was found to have deteriorated in quality – almost certainly as a result of overuse and overgrazing. Analysis of human skeletons suggested life had gone from easy to hard. There had been dramatic changes in both the environment and human health.

The invention of agriculture and the domestication of animals happened more or less simultaneously around the world. Agriculture undoubtedly produced more food for more people, but the domestication of animals also brought people into closer contact with the pathogens carried naturally by other species. As US medical historian and paleo-pathologist Ethne Barnes has written: 'The twin, irreversible agricultural and microbial revolutions were under way.'[3]

Why humans, after 200,000 or more years of reasonably successful living, should have switched in only a few hundred years from a healthy way of life to a more onerous and risky existence, growing a narrow range of crops and managing animals, has baffled historians. Theories range from climate change, population pressure and overhunting to malnutrition, migrations and disease among wild animals. It's possible, too, that people were forced to settle and farm by new power structures.

'[It is] a fundamental question to which we have no good answer,' says Mithen. 'Was it by choice or was that first sowing of seed a trap, locking people into a seasonal cycle of planting and harvesting from which we have been unable to escape?'[4]

US plant explorer, geneticist and agronomist Jack Harlan pondered the same question in 1992: 'Why farm? Why give up the 20-hour working week and the fun of hunting in order to toil in the sun? Why work harder for food less nutritious and a supply more capricious? Why invite famine, plague, pestilence, and crowded living conditions?'[5]

The old consensus was that people had eked out an existence through hunting and foraging what they could, but then happily settled down to farm and rear animals – at which point, the story goes, food surpluses started to appear, cities grew, people had leisure time and became healthier, the arts flourished and new technologies developed. Humanity, the story went, arrived healthy, more or less civilised and fully formed.

The reality was very different.

* * *

If anyone is responsible for changing the way we understand how disease evolved it may be bone detective and medical anthropologist George Armelagos. The son of Greek immigrants who came to the US in the 1930s, this genial man spent a lifetime inspecting every crevice, scratch, pit, malformation, blemish, cut and fissure in old human skeletons. He and colleagues at the University of Massachusetts ditched the old Victorian idea which held that the arrival of farming and the growth of cities improved peoples' health. When they studied nearly 600 skeletons of Native Americans in 1,000-year-old burial mounds in what are now the Ohio and Illinois river valleys, they found physically large people showing few signs of disease.

It was only when the Native Americans had started growing corn (maize) intensively around 900 years ago that health problems became evident; at this point, he says, the skeletons began to show stunting and disease. Foragers generally had excellent teeth and were rarely malnourished; they were taller than most people are today and, by and large, didn't suffer from endemic diseases or epidemics. By contrast, when Native Americans started farming crops intensively, illnesses became common and diseases like tuberculosis (TB) became established. It was around then that populations started suffering from yaws and syphilis and two-thirds showed signs of degenerative bone disease.

But even Armelagos was surprised when he and his colleagues found in 2005 that Nubians living in what is now southern Egypt and Sudan had mastered the use of antibiotics and were living a remarkably disease-free life 1,500 years before Alexander Fleming discovered modern-day penicillin and ushered in the twentieth-century revolution in healthcare. Analysis of the Nubian skeletons showed that they were saturated with tetracycline, an antibiotic first used commercially in 1978 and now used to treat malaria, plague, cholera and syphilis.

* * *

Evidence that pre-industrial peoples were fundamentally healthy comes from all over the world. A 2003 study by Durham University archaeologists of nearly 35,000 skeletons from more than 300 sites in Britain dating from 10,500 BC to AD 1850 showed that as people became sedentary, gave up their hunter-gatherer way of life and started to farm, diets became less varied and disease increased.[6] The reasons are not hard to understand. Sedentary people who grow crops manipulate the environment, cut down trees, drain swamps, hunt out some animals and introduce new ones. With these environmental changes comes the space for new pathogens to thrive and others to disappear. Each age creates the ecological conditions for its own diseases to emerge and flourish. Disease, in other words, is rooted in the environments that humans create by farming, building, burning, digging and draining.

In Africa as elsewhere, says University of Oregon medical historian Melissa Graboyes, diseases are particularly sensitive to environmental change:

> One of the biggest shifts during the past millennium [there]
> is that people's relationship to the land has changed. Until
> 5,000 BC, Africa's population was composed primarily of small
> nomadic groups engaged in hunting and gathering. These small
> groups of people travelled from place to place, hunting and
> collecting wild grains. They moved to a new location when
> the seasons changed or when a place no longer provided food.

Although it goes against many people's expectations, the disease burden was actually quite low for these nomadic people.[7]

Graboyes has shown that Africa was never the diseased continent it is often portrayed as being today. There were many things people did not have, like permanent homes or iron tools, but they also did not have many diseases common in Africa today. Waterborne diseases such as dysentery and cholera were virtually unknown, since groups would move before fouling their water supply. Their lack of contact with livestock also protected them against diseases such as smallpox or measles.[8]

Most modern human infectious diseases would probably have been unknown to our hunter-gatherer ancestors. Until about 10,000 years ago, the human population is thought to have had excellent general health, consisting almost entirely of small, nomadic groups which would have dodged infectious diseases because of their physical isolation and their limited size, which did not allow infections to spread far.[9]

Trouble began when agriculture was intensified, people started living close to each other in cities and long-distance trade developed, meaning that infections could travel further. Planting fields and tending animals may have increased populations but it created the perfect conditions for dangerous pathogens to emerge and pandemics to spread.

The hunter-gatherers of Abu Hureyra or ancient Europe, China, India and elsewhere would have been bitten by insects and suffered sporadic zoonotic diseases such as tetanus, parasitic diseases like trichinosis from roundworms, as well as some skin diseases, and head and body lice and wounds inflicted by animals, but their diseases may not have spread far or beyond their often small, isolated groups.

Sedentary agriculture, says Barnes, 'stirred up the balance between human beings and microbes' and changed both the physical environment people lived in and the microbial mix in human bodies. 'When neolithic people started to farm and live in larger groups, they unwittingly created the conditions for new interactions between humans and other organisms. It revolutionized human health.'[10]

American geographer and historian Jared Diamond summed it up well: 'Hunter-gatherers practiced the most successful and longest-lasting lifestyle in human history. In contrast, we're still struggling with the mess into which agriculture has tumbled us, and it's unclear whether we can solve it.'[11]

* * *

If Abu Hureyra is one place where people evolved from hunting and collecting wild food to growing it and rearing animals, Çatalhöyük, 3,000 years younger but only about 500 kilometres to the north in what is today Anatolia in southern Turkey, is where people were first found to live much as we do today – in large numbers and close together. Now an archaeological megasite spread over thirteen hectares and overlooking the great Konya plain, this ruin has been described as the world's first recognisable city.

If farming animals set up the conditions in which diseases could emerge, cities were the perfect place for viruses and pathogens to spread. Here in Çatalhöyük, between 9,000 and 7,000 years ago, up to 8,000 people lived in back-to-back, densely packed houses, eating early varieties of wheat, barley and vegetables, and keeping sheep and goats. There were still wild animals to be hunted and the seeds and bones of apples, almonds, fish and birds suggest people had a rich, varied diet.

Çatalhöyük, says anthropologist and author John Reader, was a 'transition' town, its people dependent on wild foods but well on their way to giving up the land and becoming urbanites with time to beautify their environments. 'Forensic and social research all suggest a healthy, egalitarian society. There is no evidence yet of the devastating epidemics that were to plague the world's cities, but the trade-off for the more sedentary life was poorer health. The many hundreds of skeletons found, often beneath the floors of the homes, show stunting and tooth decay, as well as osteoarthritis suggesting manual work, a diet of grains and people having to travel longer distances to find scarcer wild animals.'[12]

Today's epidemiologists would expect that the crowded living conditions and the size of the city inevitably helped spread diseases around, but there seem to have been few contagious diseases circulating. Reader agrees: the Neolithic people of Çatalhöyük may have had the best of all worlds, he writes.[13]

But mystery still surrounds Çatalhöyük. Why should so many people choose to live here, far from the coast, on no obvious trade route? Did these Neolithic people switch to herding animals and developing crops like lentils, peas and barley because they had a surplus of food, or because there was too little for all? The city's relative isolation may have protected it from outside pathogens and disease, but how come it flourished so early and was then abandoned, even as many other cities were starting to emerge in the Fertile Crescent some 7,700 years ago?

'All that is known is that within centuries of the demise of Çatalhöyük,' the anthropologist and Assyriologist Gwendolyn Leick writes, 'the seeds of the great Sumerian civilisations and the world's first great city states were being planted 1,500 kilometres away south of what is now Baghdad in southern Iraq.'[14]

Here in Mesopotamia, which translates as 'between the rivers', highly sophisticated empires like Eridu, Uruk, Nippur, Nineveh, Babylon and Kish all rose and fell, and disease flourished. In a burst of phenomenal creativity and change, a fully fledged urban culture emerged, inventing writing, mathematics, astrology, monumental architecture and the wheel, as well as bureaucracy. Great networks of irrigation canals enabled more food to be grown, fields were ploughed with oxen and donkeys, and cattle, sheep, goats and other animals were widely domesticated.

The city was evolving but so were microbes. These first great Middle Eastern cities would inevitably have created human and animal waste, attracting disease-carrying rats and mice, birds and insects. The more intensive farming needed to feed the growing human populations required forests to be cut down, rivers to be altered, land to be irrigated and marshes to be drained, all of which encouraged new insects and pathogens.

Storing food would have attracted flies, mites, mosquitoes, spiders, birds, reptiles and rodents, and when people came into closer contact with live and dead animals, infectious diseases would inevitably have jumped the species barrier. Stagnant water in irrigation canals would have made a good breeding ground for worms and insects that transmitted diseases such as malaria and sleeping sickness; soldiers returning from wars and merchants would have unwittingly imported new diseases and pathogens to biologically defenceless populations. The new human-made environments resulted in new human-made diseases.

These urban environments were perfect incubators for bacterial, viral, fungal and parasitic pathogens to spread and ultimately reach endemic levels. Mumps possibly evolved from people keeping wild birds and poultry, diphtheria from cattle, measles from dogs, while rubella, chickenpox and whooping cough almost certainly emerged with the rise of cities in North Africa and the Fertile Crescent. Brucellosis is thought to have started with the drinking of goat milk, and typhoid from contaminated food.

Many of these ancient diseases are still familiar. Respiratory viruses like the common cold, which possibly came from horses, and influenza, which has been linked to the domestication of ducks and waterfowl, routinely circulate and evolve into new strains that are with us today.

'The advent of farming and cities was the great accelerator of both environmental degradation and human disease,' says Mithen. 'Virtually every infectious disease ... has arisen in the last 10,000 years as an effect of civilisation: cholera, smallpox, measles, flu, chickenpox and perhaps malaria. Germs travelled with trade and people, accompanying armies, slaves or annexed peasants as they moved from state to state.'[15]

Diseases could destroy a harvest or a population of livestock, as could droughts and floods, he says. 'The frequency of flooding increased as a result of the deforestation caused by an insatiable demand for timber and fuel, and excessive grazing by goats. In the absence of trees, less rainwater penetrated the soil and reached the aquifers beneath; with deforestation came soil erosion, and with excessive irrigation came salinization and a decrease in fertility.'[16]

And with degraded lands came hunger and disease.

* * *

Evidence of early urban disease comes from 2,500-year-old Mesopotamian and Egyptian texts, biblical tablets and sacred Indian and Chinese manuscripts. Interpreted by modern physicians, they suggest that ailments like meningitis, dysentery, rheumatism, mental illness, fevers, gangrene, diarrhoea, epilepsy and possibly malaria, smallpox and bilharzia were all known 5,000 or more years ago.

Disease historian Donald R. Hopkins has traced smallpox back to well before the Christian era in Egypt, China and India.[17] In a precursor to English country doctor Edward Jenner's eighteenth-century practice of inoculating people against disease, Brahmin priests travelling the Indian countryside at least 2,000 years ago would reportedly advise people to inhale the dried scabs of smallpox sufferers, so inducing a mild form of the disease.

The Old Testament, some of which was written down 3,500 years ago, also provides clues. Scholars have found sixty-eight references to plagues and pestilences of animals, crops and people.[18] Moses and others mention 'sores that break into pustules on man and beast', 'fatal visitations' that wipe out armies and illnesses that first strike young children (Exodus 9:9). The ten great plagues of Egypt have been interpreted by some modern ecologists as linked to climate, pollution and the diseases of childhood. The Book of Revelation, traditionally dated to about AD 100, talks of pestilence as one of the signs of Judgement Day.

By the end of the Neolithic period, around 2,500–3,500 BC, the microbial world had changed irrevocably. Trade was developing between the cities of Asia, Europe and India, populations were becoming sedentary, and humans were in ever closer contact with animals.

Ethne Barnes sums it up beautifully: 'The microbial pot was being stirred with increasing vigour and disease patterns changed with each new human venture.'[19] Or, as John Reader observes: 'Infectious diseases ... are the price humanity has paid for the decision to live in large complex and densely populated urban centres.'[20] All in all, civilisation had many pluses, but it was clearly bad for your health.

* * *

When Abu Hureyra was abandoned about 8,000 years ago, the global population was possibly 8 million people; by the start of the Christian era it was 300 million. Cities had enabled a population explosion. By then, they were flourishing in China, Latin America, Europe, Africa and India, and urban populations could expect sickness to strike hard and regularly.

By the start of the Christian era, epidemics of vicious fevers, wasting diseases, worms and rashes regularly swept European and Middle Eastern cities, killing populations massively, gruesomely and in waves. Termed 'plagues' and 'pestilences', these illnesses were said by priests to have been sent by the gods to punish the sinful. Few people remotely understood where they came from. 'Plague' was quite likely a general term covering what we would now understand to be typhoid, smallpox, influenza – many different diseases. Others may never be identified.

More than thirty pathogens including anthrax, Lassa fever, scarlet fever, tuberculosis, even Ebola, have been proposed by researchers as the cause of what has become known as the Plague of Athens, which killed 75–100,000 people between 430 and 426 BC, and is said by some scholars to have contributed to the fall of classical Greece. The Athenian historian Thucydides, who was infected but survived, reported high fevers, blistered skin, vomiting and diarrhoea. It could have been Ebola or just about anything else:

> People in good health were all of a sudden attacked by violent heats in the head, and redness and inflammation in the eyes, the inward parts, such as the throat or tongue, becoming bloody and emitting an unnatural and fetid breath. These symptoms were followed by sneezing and hoarseness, after which the pain soon reached the chest, and produced a hard

cough. When it fixed in the stomach, it upset it; and discharges of bile of every kind named by physicians ensued, accompanied by very great distress.[21]

Recent genetic investigations of the teeth of a young Athenian girl who died in the epidemic and was buried in a mass grave point to typhoid, which had probably arrived on a boat from Egypt. Whatever it was, it swirled around the Mediterranean for several years, killing tens of thousands of people before fizzling out.

Medical historians see a change around the start of the Christian era. Juan Peset, the great Spanish doctor executed in 1941 by Franco after the Spanish civil war, tells how malaria was endemic in marshy areas close to cities around the world by 400 BC. 'By the fourth century BC malaria had [been established] in marshy areas where the water and crops provided the conditions for the mosquito to infect man. Evidence ... is found in Chinese, Indian, Sumerian, Assyrian, Babylonian and Egyptian cultures. The link is mentioned in the Papyrus of Ebers, dating from 1570 BC. The connection between fever and marshy areas appears in the Hippocratic text "On Airs, Waters and Places".[22]

Peset argued that the first great plague epidemic cycle started around the start of the Christian era. '[Until then] there was a rough equilibrium between human beings, cities and parasites. [Then the] equilibrium breaks down with the advent of the convoys that bring the two healthiest extremes into contact, namely China and Rome. Soldiers and merchants, animals and merchandise, slaves and prisoners all contribute to the linking up of the known world.'[23]

The Plague of Justinian, which lasted eight years (AD 541–49), may have been the first and deadliest of all the world's pandemics, killing as much as half of the population of Europe, the Middle East and Arabia. *Yersinia pestis*, the same bacterium responsible for the Black Death (1347–51), was to be the precursor of waves of plague that continued far beyond the fourteenth century.

Plagues were varied, common and unpredictable, regarded as part of the divine plan for man. Francis Leneghan, professor of Old English at Oxford, tells how it lingered for generations. 'In the sixth century, a plague spread from Egypt to Europe and lingered for the next 200 years. At the end of the seventh century, the Irish scholar Adomnán, Abbot of Iona, wrote in book 42 of his Life of St Columba of "the great mortality which twice in our time has ravaged a large part of the world".[24]

Between outbreaks of the bubonic plague came other diseases. Smallpox was unknown in Europe when it reached Italy in AD 165 at the height of Roman power. Possibly brought by troops returning from wars in the Middle East, what is now known as the Antonine plague ravaged the Roman aristocracy, depopulated cities and, by draining the coffers of the state and weakening the military, almost certainly hastened the fall of the greatest empire history had known. By the end of the outbreak in AD 180, nearly one in three people in the cities and villages affected had died.[25]

Professor W. J. MacLennan, of the Edinburgh Royal Infirmary, describes graphically how the cramped streets and buildings of Edinburgh enabled disease to spread and acted as an 'incubator' for diseases like plague to keep returning in the Middle Ages.

> Wave after wave [of plague] ... almost destroyed the rat
> and lice-infested city between the fourteenth and sixteenth
> centuries. Following a poultry disease in 1335 which forced the
> slaughter of every chicken and turkey in Scotland, there were
> severe outbreaks of human plague in 1336, 1349, 1361 and 1379,
> followed by seven more between 1498 and 1597. At one time,
> more than half the population of the city died, and people
> regularly fled to the Highlands. Those left were subject to
> curfews and ever harsher regulations to prevent the spread of
> disease. Licences were required for people to be allowed to visit
> each other, children were not allowed to play outdoors ...[26]

* * *

Even as Europe was building up some ancestral immunity to the succession of diseases that had ravaged them for centuries, the greatest ever biological and environmental change the world had known in tens of thousands of years was striking the New World, as

European countries vied to invade the Americas, taking with them their most powerful allies – disease and oppression.

It was Columbus, the fifteenth-century Portuguese colonialist and slave trader, who set in motion what may be the fastest and greatest exchange of people, animals and microbes that the world has ever seen. Within about a hundred years of his first voyage with colonists to the Caribbean in 1492, dozens of diseases that had long ravaged Europe, Asia and North Africa had been introduced to biologically defenceless Amerindian populations by adventurers, slave traders, missionaries and colonists. Wave after wave of pandemics weakened native populations in the Pacific, Australia and Southern Africa to the point where they could not resist the invasion of their lands. Far more people were to die from European diseases than would ever die by Spanish, Portuguese or British swords.

Infection possibly happened unknowingly, at least at first. Along with domesticated pigs, horses and sheep, vegetables, sugar cane and other plants, the first colonists to the Americas took with them a host of human, plant and animal pathogens that had previously been confined to Europe and Africa. When on Columbus's second voyage an anonymous crewman infected with a mild form of smallpox passed it to an indigenous American, this marked the start of the mixing of Native American, African and European pathogens and could be said to have fatally changed the world.[27]

Columbus's fourth voyage in 1502 may well have led to the introduction of malaria to the Americas, says Noble David Cook, professor of history at Florida International University, in his book *Born to Die*. 'Many of the first expeditions carried *Vivax malaria*, endemic in Mediterranean Spain, in their blood. From mid 1502 until April 1503, the men of Columbus coasted Mesoamerica. Mosquitoes were so abundant there that one section of the mainland came to be known as the Mosquito Coast.'[28]

The triangular slave trade in gold, humans and pathogens quickly developed into a vortex of misery, displacement and disease. Right from the start of his travels to the Americas in 1492, Columbus needed slaves to make the first colonies work; equally, the Spanish military who accompanied him were helped by disease to defeat the indigenous populations. The pathogens and viruses that were let loose thrived in the new, defenceless Native American hosts.

No one knows who brought falciparum malaria, the most dangerous type of malaria, to what is now Latin America and the Southern US. Cook says that it was quite likely to have been European slave traders. Malaria of any kind was completely absent from North America until Europeans arrived and was known only in a mild form in the Caribbean and South America before colonisation. But as soon as falciparum arrived it took a heavy toll with a succession of epidemics that badly affected both Europeans and indigenous peoples who had no resistance.

Within twenty years of Columbus's fourth voyage, Spanish, French and other European powers were building forts and trading stations, and rounding up West African slaves to work on the plantations and in the mines of their new European colonies. By 1520, there were possibly twenty sugar plantations using slaves on Hispaniola (modern-day Haiti/Dominican Republic) alone. By that time the indigenous Amerindian populations of most Caribbean islands had been decimated by disease and tens of thousands of hectares of virgin forest had been cleared by slaves to provide the land for more plantations. It was biological warfare on a grand scale.[29]

As the twin slave and sugar trades developed into a giant industry, so Old World diseases mutated and spread to every corner of the Western world. Over the course of 400 years, more than 10 million Africans were enslaved, more than half the world was colonised and at least thirty infectious diseases were introduced by European colonists, including influenza, measles, the plague, cholera, diphtheria, typhus, chickenpox and yellow fever. Together they were more catastrophic than the Black Death in medieval Europe, which has been estimated to have killed 25 million people.[30]

But while native populations were being decimated, the invaders more or less escaped New World diseases, thanks to the immunity they had acquired to the animal pathogens they had brought with them. Europe had developed very differently from the Americas, and its more settled farming and urban populations had long been exposed and built up some immunity to common diseases passed from domesticated livestock over millennia. Wars and international trade, too, would have exposed people to many diseases of Africa and Asia.

The Caribbean and Southern American plantations to which the slaves were transported were the breeding ground of yet more disease. Both Europeans and Africans suffered from lung, liver and bowel complaints as well as frequent fevers, but while bacteria and viruses did not distinguish between black, white and indigenous peoples, just as with Covid-19, it was the poorest and those living in the worst conditions – in this case invariably the enslaved – who fared worst.

The whole sugar plantation economy was built round disease and violence. Badly built, overcrowded housing without sanitation or clean water led to infection, malnutrition and early deaths. As the trade grew, so slave fertility declined, and planters found it cheaper to buy new slaves from Atlantic traders than to try to cure or care for diseased people. How many indigenous Mexicans, Hondurans, Bolivians, Chileans, North Americans, Brazilians and others also died from the diseases shipped from Europe to the Americas can only be guessed at. Was it 20 million? Thirty million? It was probably far, far more, says Florentine scholar Massimo Livi-Bacci.[31]

Crucially, disease accompanied the ecological destruction involved in setting up plantations. The great cotton and cane fields of the Southern American states, and Caribbean islands like Barbados and Jamaica, transformed the environment. Europeans reaching the Caribbean in the fifteenth century told of deep jungle and scrublands interspersed with clearings occupied by groups of native peoples. Three hundred years of colonialism saw river valleys cleared of trees, massive soil erosion, decimated wildlife and hillsides made bare. European settlers systematically exhausted the best lands, leaving hotspots of disease in large, chaotic townships of impoverished rural people. In less than a hundred years, writes Roger G. Kennedy, who directed the US National Park Service and the Smithsonian Institution's National Museum of American History, Amerindians were weakened by European diseases and then driven off the land to make way for Africans.[32]

When slavery ended in Haiti, the hills had been cleared of trees. The freed slaves rejected the plantation model of farming and opted for subsistence farming. This led to a population explosion and a rush to clear the best new land. Just as today's palm oil and rubber plantations in Indonesia are carved out of lush forest and provide all the conditions for infectious diseases to emerge and spill over to humans, so the clearing of Caribbean lands led to infestations of rats and mosquitoes and new human, crop and animal diseases.

2

WHAT WE KNOW NOW

On the evening of 21 September 1998, Hurricane Georges battered Puerto Rico with wind speeds of more than 115 mph, destroying nearly 30,000 homes, killing many people and causing billions of dollars' worth of physical damage.[1] It was a regional disaster which took many Caribbean islands years to recover from, but for British zoologist Kate Jones, then in her early twenties, it provided a unique chance to research the effects of extreme weather on nature and specifically on the bats she was studying. One year later, she headed for Puerto Rico's network of huge underground caverns, which were known to house some of the largest bat colonies in the world – as well as thousands of boa constrictors, which feed on the bats as they emerge at night.

Observing wildlife in the tropics was Jones's childhood dream. As a girl in the 1980s, she had fallen in love with Harrison Ford playing Dr Henry Walton 'Indiana' Jones, the fictional professor of archaeology in Hollywood's *Raiders of the Lost Ark*. She had imagined herself as an adventurer like him, travelling the world in search of exotic, even dangerous, animals. Wasn't Indiana Jones a doctor? Did they not share a family name?

Working in Puerto Rico's stinking, stifling bat- and snake-infested caves may not have proved quite as romantic as she had imagined, but she could console herself it was important, if grim, scientific work, which showed how the hurricane had indeed devastated bat populations. It also gave her an early lesson in the evolution of human disease, one which was to change her life. While in the caves she breathed in the spores of a fungus found in bat droppings and contracted a sometimes fatal infection called histoplasmosis. She recovered, but although she still loves and studies bats, her lungs were permanently damaged and she is prone to pneumonia.

Now a professor of ecology and biodiversity at University College London, she is an ebullient and popular figure, known for pursuing ambitious research projects, and called 'Cocktail Kate' by her colleagues for her ability to mix drinks. Bats spread some of the world's most dangerous diseases like Ebola and SARS, she says, but far from being the dark, mysterious and dangerous creatures of myth, they are the commonest type of mammal on earth, making up as many as 1,400, or one in five, of all known mammal species. In a series of interviews, she tells me that they should be ranked with bees as important pollinators of fruit, great dispersers of seeds and natural controllers of insects. Some do harbour deadly viruses, she accepts, but so does every mammal, and bats are no worse for viruses, species for species, than most other mammals. 'Humans cannot do without them. They changed my world and they changed the world in a positive way,' she says.

Jones and her team of researchers are part of a growing number of disease ecologists looking for patterns in the origins and spread of disease and laying the foundations of a new understanding of the connections between human health and the environment. Twenty years ago the role of biodiversity in the transmission of pathogens was poorly understood, if only because most medical scientists focused on individual conditions and ailments. Wildlife diseases, in contrast, were considered important only when they affected farming or human health, and vets and human disease researchers did not talk much to each other.

For ecologist Thomas Gillespie at Emory University in Atlanta, Georgia, who works with primates, bats and rodents in equatorial Africa, it was dramatic diseases like HIV/Aids and Ebola in the 1990s which changed the way we understand how diseases can emerge from disturbed landscapes. In an interview in 2021 he told me: 'They captured attention. It was seeing that they were linked to wildlife which was so important. We began to understand that pathogens and zoonoses – diseases passed to humans from animals – are far more common than was thought.'

As it had been for Kate Jones, his own introduction to zoonotic disease was shocking. He told me: 'I was twenty-one, I had gone out on an expedition to the Amazon and a colleague went down with cerebral malaria. He died. A few years later I went to Indonesia and caught a near fatal dose of hemorrhagic dengue fever.'

Even as I was in Mayibout 2 in Gabon, researchers like Jones and Gillespie were beginning to identify the common cause of many human infectious diseases as the disturbance of nature on both the local and planetary scale. The emerging hypothesis was simple enough, if controversial: when the environment changes – as it does when a tropical forest is felled or a landscape is heavily degraded, or the temperature increases with global warming, or animals are crowded closely together in intensive farms – then a new set of relationships between life-forms is established and animals and humans are exposed to pathogens to which they may not yet have adapted. These 'spillovers' of pathogens from one species to another mostly meet dead ends, burn out and have little effect on the emergence of disease. But very occasionally they don't – which is when pandemics and disease outbreaks mostly emerge. Escalating human and animal numbers and the dense conditions in which farm animals live, and the equally dense conditions in which humans are packed in cities, make the perfect conditions for disease to spread.

As evidence of the human impact on earth has grown, so too have the links between the diseases of animals and those of humans. The interaction between humans, their billions of domesticated animals and wildlife is now understood to be the cause of many emerging diseases. Wildlife species like birds and bats are increasingly found to be the reservoirs of the pathogens infecting domesticated farm animals like poultry; poultry and cattle are in turn passing diseases like brucellosis and bird flu to humans, and, in a process called 'reverse zoonosis', humans are being found to be transmitting infections including Covid-19, herpes and tuberculosis back to domesticated animals and pets.[2] Ancient diseases like TB, indeed, may have co-evolved between humans and animals over hundreds of thousands of years. Humans, it is found, are far from alone in experiencing pandemics. Mass die-offs of amphibians, bees, fish, birds, marine invertebrates, primates, pigs and wild dogs are all being increasingly recorded.[3]

Over twenty years, Jones, Gillespie and this new generation of disease ecologists have led research into the changing nature of disease. In a series of papers in major scientific journals they have shown how rapid human population growth and the shrinking of wildlife habitats is now driving the emergence of new diseases like HIV/Aids and Ebola.

It was a landmark study in 2000 by British wildlife ecologist Peter Daszak which set Jones and other scientists thinking about how the destruction and degradation of nature on a planetary scale might be causing many disease outbreaks. To test their hypothesis, they needed to establish whether infectious diseases were on the rise.[4] Using national medical records from every country, they researched the origins of 335 human infectious diseases known to have emerged between 1940 and 2004. In 2008, they published their landmark paper, which showed conclusively that most human infectious diseases now originated from viruses, bacteria, parasites and fungi which naturally live in wild and domesticated animals.[5]

It barely troubled the medical world but had a great influence on other researchers now delving into the relationships between biodiversity, land use and emerging infectious diseases. Jones followed it up by showing that the total number of outbreaks of infectious disease worldwide had increased steadily for the past forty years,[6] and that the variety of outbreaks had also increased significantly since 1980.[7]

Today it is widely accepted that three out of every four new or emerging infectious diseases in people come from animals and that the number of diseases jumping from animals to humans is continuing to rise. In any one month, several thousand outbreaks of disease are now recorded by global data maps.[8]

* * *

For Jones, though, the underlying causes of disease transmission from animals is rooted deeply in our destruction of ecosystems and exploitation of wild species and places. 'We have got far more people, and more densely packed populations which are moving around more. We've also got hugely fragmented landscapes because we are building lots of roads, and lots of pollution to disrupt ecosystems. We are changing land use on a global scale and it's happening at a really rapid rate. It's impacting lots and lots of different species. We are developing a changing landscape.'[9]

She and others now go further, showing how the loss of nature doesn't just result in fewer species but tends to help smaller mammals and insects, like ticks, fleas and rats, which mostly carry disease. Moreover, the populations of species known to carry diseases transmissible to humans generally increase as the landscape changes from natural to farmed and urban: 'The changes we are making to the planet don't just affect animals but have a direct impact on us, too', she says.

Nor is it just large-scale changes to the natural environment, like deforestation and urbanisation, which are encouraging diseases to emerge. Just as important are social and political factors. The industrialisation of our food system, concentrations of poverty, the spread of cities and the tripling of the world's population in just seventy-five years have all played a part.

Today there is a complete A–Z of infectious diseases known to be emerging from animals. Since HIV/Aids was first detected in 1981, the US alone has had outbreaks of more than a hundred, including chikungunya, hantaviruses, MERS, Nipah, SARS, Marburg, Lassa fever, Yersinia, Q, Valley and Zika. All are potentially lethal and most have surfaced in the US in the last twenty years.[10]

Some, like Babesia, Bartonella and Ehrlichiosis, are spread by bats and ticks and remain obscure, while new bacterial superbugs and rare fungal infections have started to appear regularly in hospitals. Most have no cures or vaccines. Individually, these new diseases are some of the nastiest imaginable. MERS attacks the nervous system.

Lyme disease dates back to the ice age in Europe but is becoming alarmingly common in North America and Europe. It has one of the longest lists of symptoms: chest pains, confusion, disturbed speech, bladder dysfunction, burning sensations, heart murmurs, paralysis, forgetfulness, the unavoidable need to sit down, hair loss, mood swings, vertigo, dizziness and more than forty others.[11]

New and old diseases can now pop up almost anywhere at any time. The World Health Organization's global disease surveillance teams report dozens of unusual disease outbreaks every month. Since 2011, there has been a dramatic 63 per cent spike in outbreaks in Africa, especially of diseases like Mpox, Ebola and dengue. 'People are coming into closer contact with animals and their pathogens as better road, rail, boat and air transport allows easier access to remote areas, but also as farming encroaches more on to the habitats of wildlife,' says Matshidiso Moeti, the WHO's regional director for Africa. 'Infections originating in animals and then jumping to humans have been happening for centuries, but the risk of mass infections and deaths has been relatively limited in Africa. Poor infrastructure acted as a natural barrier.'[12]

Infectious disease outbreaks may still be rare in rich and middle-income countries, but as the gap between rich and poor grows, they are becoming more common in the world's developing countries. To get an idea of the scale, I searched the database for March 2020. Even as Covid-19 was starting to spread round the world, a new mosquito-borne dengue fever epidemic was hitting Afghanistan, yellow fever was rampant in Mali, there was Mpox in Singapore, cholera appeared in Somalia, Crimean-Congo hemorrhagic fever surfaced in Pakistan, typhoid arrived in Fiji and MERS hit Saudi Arabia. In addition, the US had its worst outbreaks of measles in twenty-five years. In the following two years, monkeypox spread to seventy-two countries, Marburg – similar to Ebola – broke out in Ghana for the first time, wild polio, thought to have been eradicated in Africa, returned to Malawi and Mozambique, and mosquito-borne chikungunya continued to explode across both Asia and Africa. Meanwhile, African swine fever was decimating pig populations around the world and avian flu was circulating in the poultry farms of more than fifty countries and in wild birds everywhere.

I asked Mark Woolhouse, professor of disease epidemiology at Edinburgh University, whether diseases were emerging more frequently, or whether we were getting better at surveillance. He called it 'chatter' – the term used by anti-terrorist squads to refer to many small events that might signify something more serious gathering on the horizon.

A remarkable shift has taken place in the diseases humans now suffer. In the past, most people everywhere died from infectious diseases. Today, most people in wealthy countries die of degenerative non-communicable diseases like cancers, heart disease, diabetes, dementia and chronic lung disease (COPD). Indeed, of all the great historical infectious diseases that plagued the world for centuries, only tuberculosis is still a major worldwide cause of death, infecting millions of people every year. It and other greatly feared diseases like typhoid, cholera, yellow fever, syphilis and gonorrhoea, thought just thirty years ago to be close to eradication, are now re-emerging strongly, especially in the world's poorest cities.

Any complacency there may have been in the late twentieth century that infectious diseases were declining has proved woefully misplaced. Age-old demons like plague and anthrax are back; malaria still kills more than a million people annually; cholera, the curse of the eighteenth century, still affects thousands of people every year and austerity and poverty-linked Victorian-era diseases like scarlet fever, gout and whooping cough are on the rise in Europe, possibly because they have adapted to antibiotic drugs and a hesitancy in people to have vaccinations.

Covid-19 was just the latest infectious disease to be linked closely to human activity. The World Health Organization estimates that one in four deaths a year, around 12 million, now come as a direct result of people's exposure to unhealthy environments. Pollution of the air and water is still the greatest killer of all but when zoonotic and other infectious diseases like malaria, schistosomiasis and dengue fever, all of which are highly sensitive to man-made changes in environmental conditions, are included, it is likely that more than half of all human deaths every year are now linked directly to the environments in which we live. Meanwhile, some diseases that until the start of the Second World War had been mostly mild, like West Nile virus, Zika and Rift Valley fever, have now crossed continents and mutated into killers.[13]

In 1996, when Ebola hit Mayibout 2, it was barely understood that climate change would reduce the amount of food grown or fundamentally change the spread of human diseases, or that the most important reservoirs of pathogens that can jump into humans are bats, rodents, primates and some birds. Twenty-five years on, it is clear that the planet's climate is on the move, affecting all species and opening a Pandora's Box of unknown pathogens which are already having immense consequences for our own health and that of all other species. Throughout history, advances in civilisation – agriculture, domestication, urbanisation and globalisation – have all been accompanied by increasing disease risk. But never before has the human population been so large, so hyper-connected and living at such high densities. We are now approaching a storm of spiralling disease risk.

Between the emergence of Ebola in 1978 and Covid-19 in 2019, a wealth of new field and laboratory research, as well as bitter experience, has taught us how disturbing habitats and reducing biodiversity profoundly changes the distribution of species and upsets the balance between them, affecting the health of animals, plants and humans. It is now accepted, too, that crowding animals or trading them in unsanitary conditions can incubate and spread disease by increasing the chances of a spillover of pathogens. Just as deforestation changes the balance of animal species in an environment, so there is now good ecological evidence to show that large-scale monocultures of trees and crops can reduce plants' resilience to pest diseases, temperature rises and droughts.[14]

Equally, we can now see clearly how humans are reducing the space for wild animals. Building dams and giant irrigation projects may help grow food or generate electricity but it also creates breeding sites for disease-carrying insects and snails; the uncontrolled growth of cities can lead to denser human populations and the faster transmission of diseases between people. Critically, a warming world is now known to be a sicker world, causing diseases of plants and animals to increase both by compromising the hosts and because many microorganisms become more virulent at warmer temperatures.

Meanwhile, increased temperatures have allowed disease-carrying insects like mosquitoes and ticks to breed more prolifically and move to new places. The world's many new biological research laboratories have increased the chances of pathogens escaping. The legal and illegal wildlife industries and the intensive farming of so many animals incubates and amplifies the risk of diseases mutating and spreading not just between farms but into human populations; the ease of travel, growth of cities and the sheer increase in the number of people living close to each other have all helped drive the emergence and spread of diseases.

We also know that new viruses are more likely to emerge in some parts of the world than others. Tropical Africa, Latin America and Asia are the hotspots because of their high biodiversity and the great environmental changes taking place there. We know, too, that new strains of disease have more chance of surfacing in crowded farms and unhygienic marketplaces where animals are crowded together.

In addition, we know that the way we grow food and encroach on other species gives pathogens, viruses and bacteria the chance to emerge, spill over into human populations and lead to infections, sometimes serious outbreaks and very occasionally pandemics. In short, we are learning that although the pathogens that cause diseases are entirely natural, humankind is creating the perfect conditions for them to emerge and spread diseases. We are learning, too, that humans, plants and animals are now in a new, closer and riskier relationship. Covid-19, as well as HIV, Ebola, bird flu, SARS and all the other infectious diseases that have emerged in the last fifty years were just the first out of the Pandora's box that we have opened.[15]

But to see how humans are driving these changes and understand how we may be able to control diseases in the coming years, we must head back to the forests.

3

THE DYING FALL

We were deep in the steaming Congolese rainforest close to Mbandanka, right on the equator line, and I had spent all day watching loggers charge around with chainsaws and small bulldozers, smashing through the undergrowth to reach giant okan, sipo, moabi, douka and iroko trees to send to wealthy countries. I'd seen pine forests being felled in Canada and Scandinavia, and ancient oaks and beeches cut down in Europe, but this was said to be 'selective' logging' of the equatorial forest and it was the most brutal I had seen.

It wasn't just the scale and speed of this logging operation, the destination of the wood or even the visual loss that was so shocking – but how much life is lost when a single big tree is felled. In this case, all the valuable and large trees across an area the size of London had been identified and were being felled for flooring, furniture, even concrete shuttering. Nothing was to be spared.

Big trees play a special role in forests. They may make up less than 2 per cent of the trees but they can contain one quarter of the total biomass and are vital for the health of the whole forest because they provide most of the seeds. With their crowns basking way above the forest canopy, they capture vast amounts of energy, which allows them to produce massive crops of fruits, flowers and foliage that sustain much of the animal life below. Their canopies help moderate the local forest environment while their understorey creates a unique habitat for other plants and animals.

Because the Democratic Republic of Congo straddles the equator, where there is the most warmth and rain, its forests are some of the most biologically rich on earth. Here, a bush may have more species of ant living in it than may live in the entire United Kingdom, and lowland gorillas, shy forest elephants, bongos, bats, hyenas and antelope may share the space with groups of indigenous peoples. Not one square metre of primary equatorial forest is uninhabited or unused by someone or some creature.

We watched Alphonse and Laurent, two young loggers each wielding a heavy-duty metre-long chainsaw, take turns to attack a massive moabi tree. These increasingly rare forest giants can grow sixty metres tall. This one was possibly 200 years old but it took no more than thirty minutes to fell. When the chainsaws stopped, the young loggers ran for their lives; the great trunk barely moved for minutes, it seemed, then creaked and ever so slowly at first and then with a great crack crashed down, taking with it smaller trees, bushes, lianas, creepers and vines. When it hit the forest floor there was a great shuddering, then a splintering of wood; then a humming and a cloud of what looked like dust rose six metres from the ground.

But it was not dust. For several minutes the stricken moabi seemed to rain birds, flies, seeds, spores, leaves, bees, flowers, wasps, nests, ants, beetles, moths, frogs, snails and all the thousands of insects and small mammals that had lived together in that tree. As their myriad homes were destroyed, so all the wildlife dependent on that tree rose in alarm. Anything that could, flew. Everything else ran, crawled, burrowed, hid or took its chances. A complete ecosystem with thousands of interdependent organisms and microorganisms had been transformed in a few moments.

When a tree like that moabi falls, hundreds of relationships between plants and creatures, plants and humans, animals and humans, and animals and animals, change. First to leave will be the birds, butterflies, moths and bats that can fly to safety. Then the mammals that use the tree for shelter or food will move deeper into the forest to seek new safe niches or hunting grounds. Last to escape – or not – are the little creatures like rats and fleas, ticks and ants, fungi, bacteria, microbes and all those creatures, pathogens and life-forms which live or depend on the soil.

And because each piece of this complex ecosystem relies upon other pieces, every change has potentially far-reaching consequences: a falling tree in a dense forest will open a clearing that will allow in sunlight and let new life flourish. A small species of frog may lose its niche in the high branches of the tree but if it perishes, then it may affect the population of a certain bird that relies on it for food and which alone disperses the seeds of a plant which in turn is used by a human. New life may benefit when normal predators disperse or as light levels change, but all life will be altered.

When whole forests are felled, as tens of thousands of square kilometres are every year in equatorial Latin America, Africa and Indonesia, the animal world cannot keep up and the ecological changes taking place are of another order. On the grandest, global scale, the deep, peaty soils in which so much of the world's tropical forest is rooted start to dry up and blow away, releasing vast amounts of CO_2, blocking waterways and reducing fertility. The ground absorbs more heat, affecting cloud formation, which in turn affects the temperature and rainfall, with the ultimate result that the conditions in which life must exist become more challenging.

But what has only lately been better understood is that ecological disruption creates the perfect conditions for new diseases and pathogens to emerge, for old ones to resurface, for dangerous ones to spill over into other species and for worldwide pandemics to occur. In short, in changing the natural world so profoundly and by altering the relationship between species so quickly, humans have become the unwitting architects of their own demise.

* * *

To better understand how the loss of biodiversity might lead to human disease I turned to Amy Vittor, who in 2009 had been one of a group of American medical researchers from Wisconsin in the US Midwest heading for the Peruvian Amazon. The question they wanted to answer was whether deforestation increased or reduced the risk of malaria. After years of debate, the jury was still out. On the one hand, there was plenty of research showing that logging and building roads in forests creates the puddles and ruts perfect for certain mosquitoes and other insects to breed. On the other, when trees are cut down and roads are paved, there are fewer breeding places and less disease.

Their destination was Iquitos, a major port thousands of kilometres up the river Amazon which had been carved out of the jungle in the late nineteenth-century rubber boom years. The city – like Manaus, almost 1,500 kilometres to the east on the banks of the Brazilian Amazon – is a world of its own, surrounded by forest and with an extraordinary vibrancy but a dark history of slavery, poverty and disease. Ever since US rubber barons enslaved local tribes and brought in West Indian labour to collect and export raw latex rubber from the forest, this city that cannot be reached by road has attracted settlers and adventurers and has been plagued with epidemics of malaria, dengue, yellow fever and more lately Zika and Covid-19. Today it has a population of about 400,000 people and some of the worst slums in Latin America, and is growing fast. In 2020 it became a global hotspot for Covid-19 and images of its overflowing hospitals and graveyards were beamed around the world.[1]

Vittor and her team arrived in Iquitos in 2009 on the heels of a major malaria epidemic that had infected as many as one in three people. This had coincided with one of the city's regular spurts of physical expansion and the arrival of many thousands of impoverished gold miners, settlers and others seeking cheap land to work and a better life. The question for the researchers was how, or if, malaria and the arrival of more people were connected. One theory was that the disease arrived and was spread by people carrying the parasite that carried the disease, who were flooding into the city; another was that these new arrivals were changing the landscape, cutting down thousands of trees to make small-scale farms.

Vittor, today a professor of infectious diseases at the University of Florida's emerging pathogen institute in Miami, embarked on an ambitious experiment to search for mosquito larvae around the Nanay river, a tributary of the Amazon. Every day she travelled about twenty kilometres out of Iquitos and, setting up fifty-six research sites with kilometre-long lines radiating from each of them, she directed teams of people to sample with nets all the many hundreds of streams, ponds and puddles along each line. Working every day and often late into the night for over a year, they tested and compared virgin, degraded and cleared forest, collecting 5,524 water samples. They identified about 24,000 mosquitoes – 'half of whom seemed to bite us', she recalls.

Not all mosquitoes carry malaria, but of those that did, a far greater number were found in the more heavily deforested landscapes. Surprisingly, though, it did not seem to matter how many people were around. In all, Vittor found malaria-carrying mosquitos in one in six of the ponds and streams where deforestation was heavy, and one in ten of the streams and rivulets where forest disturbance was light, but in only one in fifty places where the water was surrounded by intact forest. It seemed pretty conclusive. They also checked with people. One in three people living near recently deforested areas or involved in logging caught the disease that year – many more than in places where the trees were still standing.[2]

Field research by Vittor and other ecologists increasingly points to landscape change as the likely source of much human disease. Cutting down trees, flooding large areas to make dams, mining and changing land use from forest to farmland all increases the risk of zoonotic – or animal-borne – diseases. Biting insects like mosquitoes, ticks, flies, fleas and bugs, all of which thrive in ecologically disturbed areas, are together associated with at least sixteen major infectious diseases, including malaria, meningitis, plague, rabies, hantavirus, yellow fever, dengue, Rift Valley fever and Lyme disease.

Vittor is one of a group of global medical disease investigators making the links between ecological disturbance and health. Her research, and that of others, increasingly shows diseases emerging when forests are fragmented as opposed to when they remain intact, and it is people living on their edges rather than deep within them who are most affected. After Peru she headed for a forested region in Panama known as Darien where more than a hundred cases of a severe, mosquito-borne neurological disease similar to South American eastern equine encephalitis virus had recently broken out in humans for the first time. She and colleagues spent a year sampling the blood of almost 600 different mammal species in the area in search of antibodies to Madariaga virus, which would signify an infection. They identified the long-whiskered rice rat as the host for the longstanding Venezuelan equine virus, and the short-tailed cane mouse as that for the new, genetically similar Madariaga. Crucially, both rodent species thrived on the edge of forests among the young trees and pasturelands that grow back after virgin forest has been cut down.

Vittor and others are now exploring the idea that viruses are more likely to transfer to humans or animals if they live in or near human-disturbed ecosystems, like recently cleared forests or swamps drained for farmland, mining projects or housing projects. What may be happening, the thinking goes, is that deforestation drives out some species from their evolutionary niches into man-made environments where they interact and breed new strains of disease. As their natural habitats shrink, to be replaced with plantations or pastureland, they are forced to concentrate into ever-smaller territories on the edges of forests where they die out or come into closer contact with humans.

'The fragmentation brings [together] people and animal species that normally would not be interacting. The more we disturb the natural environment the more we are shaking the [microbial] pot. The links are becoming clear that disturbance leads to downstream emergence events in humans,' Vittor says.[3]

Writing with Gabriel Laporta, a Brazilian virologist with whom she has worked, Vittor argues:

These leaps from animals, or insects, to humans often happen at the edges of the world's tropical forests. Yellow fever, malaria, Venezuelan equine encephalitis, Ebola – all of these pathogens

occur at the margins of forests … As the forest is degraded
bit by bit, animals still living in isolated fragments of natural
vegetation struggle to survive. But when human settlements
encroach on these forests, human–wildlife contact can increase,
and new opportunistic animals may also migrate in. The
resulting disease spread shows the interconnectedness of natural
habitats, the animals that dwell within it, and humans.[4]

Some of the most significant research linking disease emergence
to deforestation has been conducted in West and Central Africa in
the wake of Ebola outbreaks since 1976. While the reservoir animal
may be an elusive bat or a primate, studies show that the deadly
virus emerges on the edges of forest lands that have been disturbed
in the previous few years.

In 2017 biologist Jesus Olivero from the University of Malaga,
John Fa from the Center for International Forestry Research and
an international team of researchers analysed the forty Ebola
outbreaks that had been reported. All but two of those for which
there was deforestation data showed that there had been significant
tree-felling nearby in the preceding two years. It looked likely, they
said, that it takes the Ebola-carrying bat about two years to migrate
to the felled area from the depths of the rainforest.

'These newly opened areas could be attractive to animals that
carry the virus. There is an association with open areas and fruit
bats,' said Fa. Curiously, every Ebola outbreak in humans has also
been the result of the introduction of a new strain of the virus from
an animal population and an outbreak has never occurred in the
same area twice. It is possible that in addition to concentrating Ebola
wildlife hosts, forest fragmentation may also serve as a corridor for
pathogen-carrying animals to spread the virus over large areas, and it
may increase human contact with these animals along the forest edge.

Vittor, Gabriel, Fa and others readily acknowledge that there is
plenty that is still not known about how specific viruses jump from
wildlife to humans and what might drive those contacts. But the
hypothesis that diseases are emerging from forest fragments and along
forest edges stands up. 'While many species disappear as forests are

cleared, others have been able to adapt. Those that adapt may become more concentrated, increasing the rate of infections,' says Vittor.[5]

* * *

I wanted to know how common disease was in societies that had learned to live largely undisturbed in forests. I had been told of a remarkable but little-known tribe called the U'wa who lived in the cloud forests of northeastern Colombia. To get to them meant crossing the plain from Bogotá, heading into the mountains, abandoning cars, taking to footpaths, fording rivers and then waiting. It could take weeks, I was told, not because the road was hard – although it was – but because the U'wa had learned above all that human outsiders bring disease. Any infection introduced into these remote indigenous communities can turn quickly into a lethal epidemic if no immunity has been built up.

The U'wa had good reason to be cautious. In the sixteenth century Spanish conquistadors had decimated their populations, first with measles, then with what was probably TB and a succession of other illnesses. Now oil companies wanted their lands, and in their cosmology oil was the blood of Mother Earth. After two weeks of being quarantined and closely observed in a small encampment at the base of their territory, word came from the mountain that we would be welcome to visit their villages. But Zizuma, the sacred heart of their territory, would be strictly off-limits and we could not meet their shamans and spiritual leaders or go to the cliff off which in the sixteenth century a group of U'wa had thrown themselves rather than be taken by the Spanish soldiers.

Instead, a sprite of a man, Betencaro, was sent to us. He led us on steep, barely used tracks into the U'wa forests, where he invited us to his home. But it took us over an hour to go the last few hundred metres, because he insisted on stopping every few steps to show us how the U'wa used every plant and tree for food or medicines and how they managed the forest, which they had lived in for centuries.

To the outsider, this part of the forest looked undisturbed. But to the U'wa, it was a carefully tended, all-in-one pharmacy, supermarket, vegetable garden and orchard. Betencaro was effusive, dashing from plant to tree: the root of this cured stomach pains, he said; the leaf of that was an anaesthetic that left the mouth numb in a few seconds. He pointed out shrubs that were good for headaches, another to cure fevers, more which were good to eat, a flower that glowed in the dark, a fruit that tasted of whipped cream.

He twisted a vine to make a sling to climb a tree and brought us down some honeycomb. Everything, from the leaves that served as plates to the poisonous plant he used to catch fish and the bark of a tree that was used as a contraceptive, was useful. He hunted deer, armadillos and tapirs, cultivated maize and a few wild vegetables, gathered nuts and fruit. Every plant and animal had a story, and was nurtured or tended for food or medicine. The forest itself could cure and provide for everyone.

Betencaro explained how his community's health and the world's – he made no distinction between them – were intertwined. The U'wa depended on nature, which in turn depended on the U'wa's protection. Yet this was no paradise of well-being, he insisted. The U'wa were far from disease or accident-free: women died in childbirth, children were bitten by snakes, they all knew stomach pains and toothaches and headaches, even strange illnesses.

But to keep themselves and the world in good health, they had learned over millennia to follow strict rules and rituals, tradition and ceremonies, like only taking fallen fruit, never cutting down certain trees, collecting and harvesting only certain wild plants, leaving some seed pods where they fell, hunting certain animals at precise times of the year and setting aside core, or sacred, areas into which only shamans were allowed. 'That way there is enough for all and no illness comes. Our role [on earth] is to protect the forest,' he told us. Each day the U'wa said they sang the world into existence. 'Without us there would be no world,' he said.

Eight hundred kilometres to the south and east over the Andes in the Brazilian heart of the greatest rainforest on earth, Davi Kopenawa, shaman, leader and chronicler of the Yanomami peoples, one of the largest tribes of the Amazon, also explained to me how wary his communities had had to become of visitors to protect themselves from disease.

The Yanomami had avoided the sixteenth-century and later Spanish and Portuguese conquistadors but their communities had been decimated by successive malaria epidemics that followed the roads being built through their territory and by the gold miners arriving in the 1980s. These diseases killed possibly one in five of his people, including his mother and an uncle. He only escaped by hiding in the forest for months to avoid the 'smoke', as he called the disease.

> Our health was always good. The problems we face all come from outsiders. In the past we had missionaries, then gold miners brought diseases to us. Malaria only existed on the outskirts of Yanomami territory. Now it is the main reason for our deaths. One in five of our people died in the 1980s after gold miners invaded villages and exposed us to diseases to which we had no immunity. Mosquitoes hit the gold miners first and then us.
>
> Before strangers arrived in the forest people did not die very often. Once in a while, a very old man or woman would pass away when their hair had become really white. At the time the forest did not know all the epidemics that came with the white people. These diseases come from very far away and the shamans do not know anything about them. We easily die of them, and today the shamans need to rely on white people's medicine to keep these new diseases from us.[6]

I met Davi twice again. In 2004 he reported that Western illnesses had ravaged the indigenous Yanomami again and again to the point where he felt they could not survive for much longer. In 2017 he came to Europe to warn that gold miners, or *garimpeiros*, were again stripping the forests and poisoning the rivers bringing disease with them.

'They [the white people] have brought other diseases to which we have no resistance. TB, skin diseases, dysentery, flu, even yellow fever and hepatitis. More than enough of us have experienced the epidemics of white people. Our people were many and in good health until suddenly all were decimated,' he told me.

By March 2021 there had been 50,000 confirmed cases of Covid-19 and over 900 deaths among Brazil's 300-odd indigenous communities, the disease reaching even the most remote groups, including the Yanomami.[7] I got a message through to Davi to ask how the communities were faring. Word came back that another tragedy was underway. The twin plagues of the white people had returned. The Yanomami environment was being trashed by miners again and disease was returning. History was repeating itself.[8]

* * *

Disentangling all the many possible causes of disease makes it hard to nail down the precise links between forests and human diseases, but there is a good example to be found in India. Back in 1957, entomologists were asked to investigate reports of the strange deaths of monkeys in the great Kyasanur Forest in the Western Ghat mountains of South India. But even as they searched for the dying animals, word came that people in some villages close to the forest were also dying from a disease with symptoms including fevers, headaches and diarrhoea.

It took nearly seventy years to understand how and why the outbreaks were occurring. In the 1950s the only disease that scientists knew could kill both monkeys and people was yellow fever, which was known to be spread by a mosquito; the disease was also very rare in India and therefore an unlikely candidate. It was only when three of the researchers themselves fell ill after handling ticks on the bodies of the dead monkeys that they found the first clue. It was identified as a deadly viral disease. The virus was isolated and the sickness was dubbed Kyasanur Forest disease (KFD) or monkey fever, and was linked to ticks.

Since 1957 the KFD virus has affected thousands of monkeys, as well as between 400 and 500 people a year, and it has killed more than 400 people. But it remains a mystery. In 2006, for some reason as yet unknown, it jumped hundreds of kilometres. There were theories that it had come from Russia, or that birds had brought it. By 2016 it had affected 9,500 people in sixteen districts and had spread to Goa.

One badly affected village was Banikkoppa in Karnataka state. Here a young farming couple, Nagaratna and Suresh, became ill in January 2014 from what they thought was flu.[9] When the fever did not subside after five days, they went to the local health centre. Eventually, blood samples were sent to the National Institute of Virology in Pune, where it was confirmed they had KFD, along with 135 other people in the area that year.[10]

Since then several studies have firmly established that many of the outbreaks are linked to deforestation.[11] The origins seem to date back to 1957, when hundreds of hectares of forest were cleared to make room for a large cashew-nut farm. At other times, infected people have been known to take their cattle into the forests to create large cashew plantations. One outbreak in Shivamogga district in 2014 could also have been linked to the clearing of 4,000 hectares of land a few years previously.[12]

I caught up with Kartik Sunagar from the Indian Institute of Science in Bangalore, who has studied KFD. In many villages, he told me, grazing cattle in unprotected forest patches is a common practice. 'People also venture into forests to collect dry leaves to make manure. This is mostly when humans contract the disease as they get bitten by ticks. Encroachment into forest land for cultivation and converting forests into pasturelands not only leads to habitat destruction but also increases human–wildlife interactions. Often, these events expose us to deadly and unencountered pathogens.'[13]

The findings of field researchers are backed by recent studies of global patterns of diseases. Kelly Austin, a researcher at Lehigh University in Pennsylvania, took data on forest cover in countries from the UN's Food and Agriculture Organization and malaria prevalence rates from the World Health Organization and overlaid them. She found that even when factoring in how good the healthcare was in each country, countries which had lost the most forest had higher rates of malaria and other mosquito-borne diseases. Changes to the natural environment, she concluded, created ideal conditions for malaria-carrying mosquitoes to breed.

Two years later, disease ecologists Andrew MacDonald from the University of California at Santa Barbara and his Stanford

University colleague Erin Mordecai analysed more than a decade of data showing the occurrences of malaria in nearly 800 villages, towns and cities across the Brazilian Amazon. They also looked at satellite-tracked deforestation over that same time frame and showed conclusively that an increase in deforestation led to an increase in disease transmission.[14]

One of the most important studies of global trends was conducted at the height of the first Covid-19 lockdown of 2020, when evolutionary ecologist Serge Morand from the French Agricultural Research Centre for International Development in Montpellier (CIRAD) and others analysed nearly 4,000 outbreaks of more than a hundred zoonotic diseases and 2,000 outbreaks of sixty-nine vector-borne infectious diseases recorded around the world between 1990 and 2016. They found that disease was closely linked not only to deforestation, but specifically to the rise in the number of plantations of soya, palm oil and other commodity crops planted to grow animal food. They proved conclusively that it was demand for meat that was causing both deforestation and epidemics of malaria, dengue and other diseases.[15]

According to Morand,

> The emergence of these epidemics is largely due to the growing role of animals – pets and livestock – in our environment. It multiplies the risk of a virus 'jumping' from one species to another, including humans, which has been the case for all of the recent pandemics. In addition, this has led to a massive loss of biodiversity. The production of vegetable proteins – soybeans, maize, etc. – to feed all of those animals encourages deforestation in South Asia, the Amazon Basin, and increasingly in Africa.

He added: 'A lesser-known consequence is that it also upsets the natural balance and resilience mechanisms that used to help us resist epidemics.'[16]

4

FEVER'S FLAMES

Mike Rogge, his wife Meghan and their three-year-old son Elliott were leaving Lake Tahoe when I caught up with them in mid-August 2021. For several weeks they had lived under hazy skies and smelt the Dixie wildfire, the biggest in California history, burning 150 kilometres away to their north and west in the Sierra Nevada mountains.

But now the giant Caldor fire had started and was ripping through the El Dorado national forest about eighty kilometres away. A hot Pacific wind was driving the smoke over the lip of the mountains down into the great basin where they lived. The sun was a dull orange, the sky dark and full of ash.

Ten years of drought had turned this rugged, heavily forested Northern California landscape into a tinderbox. By Friday 17 August, the Caldor fire was doubling in size every few days and smoke was building up in Lake Tahoe city. The pristine cobalt-blue lake and its surrounding mountains, a mecca for both winter skiers and summer tourists and hikers, was shrouded in mist. Now the peaks were invisible and the air quality, as registered by the official monitors, showed 250 and rising – officially unhealthy and requiring respirators or masks. They decided to stay at home. Mike went to the local hardware store, bought tape and sealed all the windows and doors to try to stop the smoke from getting in. It helped but not that much. They started wearing their Covid masks indoors.

On Tuesday 21 August the winds shifted and the smoke around Lake Tahoe thickened. The Pollock fire in 2020 had briefly registered over 200 on the international air pollution index in Tahoe but the Caldor was by now one of the worst fires in California's recorded history and moving inexorably towards them.

When they went to bed that night the closest flames were around seventy kilometres away and the air monitor read just under 400 – officially 'hazardous'. When they woke up Caldor was fifteen kilometres closer and reading 530 – or well over forty times the World Health Organization's recommended safe level. Other communities around the lake were peaking at over 600, and one, on the north shore of the lake, registered 762 – by far the highest in the US that day. The *LA Times* said the air quality in Tahoe that day was 'possibly' the worst in the world.

There was still no order to evacuate and no immediate danger of their house catching fire but Mike and Meghan had had enough. That morning, as a dense orange haze blanketed the whole area and they started to cough and fear for little Elliott, they hurriedly packed their most important belongings, got in their camper van and joined the cars beginning to leave Tahoe.

'Time to go. AQI is too high. We're heading south. Send your best wishes, prayers, vibes to our firefighters,' Mike tweeted, as the family set off on a five-hour drive to friends.

* * *

Even as the Rogges were leaving Tahoe, firefighters were trying to save villages and communities 3,000 kilometres away in Siberia with shovels, hoes and anything they could find to dampen the flames. Turbo-charged by month-long heatwaves, some of the largest wildfires and densest smoke ever recorded in the region had already burned through 13 million hectares of the great boreal forest and the fires were still advancing. The whole semi-autonomous Yakutia region in the far east of Russia was engulfed in thick smoke and there was no end in sight of the longest drought ever recorded there.

The smoke from both the Siberian and Californian megafires could be seen that day from 600 kilometres above earth on

NASA's Terra satellite.[1] Pulled by the jet stream, the Russian smoke had already wafted 3,200 kilometres east to west and 4,000 north to south, drifting over the North Pole into Canada and circumnavigating the northern hemisphere.

That August day the whole world seemed wreathed in smoke. The EU was reporting major fires raging in Greece, Bulgaria, Turkey, Italy, Albania and Spain. Southern Europe, said the Reuters news agency, had turned into a wildfire 'hotspot', with temperatures reaching record levels of over 45°C in Sicily. But the fires in Siberia were said to be larger than the ongoing fires in Greece, Turkey, Italy, the US and Canada combined.

Meanwhile, in the southern hemisphere, the NASA satellite picked up a thick shroud of smoke from hundreds of fires burning in Paraguay and southern Brazil,[2] blowing southeastward and covering, according to the NASA Worldview app, more than 274,000 square kilometres. In the Brazilian Amazon, hundreds of fires were burning following recent illegal deforestation.

The summer of 2021 may be remembered for its orange skies and vast smoke clouds,[3] but continental-scale smoke clouds have been known for years. One, in the Peace River district of Northern British Columbia in Alberta, Canada, in 1950, reportedly choked the entire northern hemisphere. In New York, where the skies were red, there were fears that an atomic bomb had been dropped; in Edinburgh, the Scots thought it was the end of the world.

Wildfire is an ever-present, natural process shaping both landscape and disease. Historically, most have been started by lightning strikes, but they happened rarely, had ecological benefits and were usually limited to a 'fire season' of a few months. But in the past thirty or so years, changes in the way land is used have altered their composition, number and duration. Human expansion into forested areas, the spread of farming deep into wild lands and the planting of forests of all one species have made wildfires both more common and more ecologically dangerous. The changes have helped accelerate global warming by increasing the vast amounts of CO_2, but they have also led to more disease and illness.

The human hand now dominates degraded landscapes. Colorado scientist Jennifer Balch, who researches the effect of fires on the world's great forests, showed in 2017 how wildfires these days are, at least in the US, nearly all human-made. She checked official records of more than 1.5 million wildfires that had to be extinguished in the US between 1992 and 2012 and found that 84 per cent of them – spreading over more than 5 million hectares – had been started by human accident or arson. Barbecues, discarded cigarettes, campfires left unattended and sparks from railways and power lines, as well as arson, all routinely caused fires, she found. Moreover, the wildfire season now stretched over five months, or three times as long as it did in the 1950s, when bush fires were mostly caused by lightning strikes.

But there was another factor. Regional warming and the drying out of fragmented forests and croplands by climate change was clearly having a major effect on wildfires but most are now also driven by anarchic, unplanned urban development and the changes in the way land is used. In North America, millions of new homes have been built close to or in forested or other 'wild' land close to cities. One 2018 study calculated that over 14 million homes were built between 1990 and 2010 in this 'wildland–urban' area.[4] Building in heavily vegetated land is what people want, but the risk of fire is greater.

Equally in Europe, large areas of farmland, especially in Mediterranean countries, have been abandoned as the economy moved to coasts, and replaced by highly flammable forest or shrublands. Former Greek finance minister Yanis Varoufakis recalls graphically the Black Monday in 2019 when more than a hundred people died when cut off by a fire outside Athens, including a friend.[5] 'The cause of the fire was obvious to anyone willing to take a disinterested look at the way a dense settlement had been inserted into an ageing pine forest with narrow lanes offering no realistic chance of escape from an inevitable inferno,' he said.[6] Similarly in Australia, the number of wildfires has increased dramatically in twenty years. Prior to 2000, there had been one megafire in Victoria in 150 years of records. But between 2002 and 2009 some

3 million hectares, or 40 per cent of the state's public land, had burned.[7]

* * *

The Rogges' snap decision to leave proved wise. By Monday 30 August, they were 800 kilometres away and the fire had moved to within thirty kilometres of Lake Tahoe. Tens of thousands of locals and tourists had been ordered to evacuate, many of the roads out of town were closed and ash was raining down on long lines of cars, some piled high with belongings and others towing trailers with bikes and other recreation equipment. The rush to leave South Lake Tahoe was becoming more chaotic by the hour.[8]

The immediate health effect of wildfires is stinging eyes and a sore throat, but the longer-term effect of smoke pollution is life-changing. No two wildfires are the same, say smoke researchers, and their health impact depends on the vegetation being burned, the weather conditions, the intensity of the fire, the moisture of the wood, the mixture of gases and toxins emitted and how long someone breathes in the smoke. There is a difference between the toxins emitted in tropical and temperate fires, and those that burn on peatlands are thought to emit tinier particles of soot.

But if smoke from natural fires is mixed with that of burning houses or cars and the plastic and the cocktail of chemicals they contain, it is certain to be far more dangerous than if a savannah grassland catches fire. To make it worse, fire departments in California are increasingly using fire retardants to spray forests and vegetation, which if breathed in or deposited on food may have their own long-term health consequences.[9]

Just as in urban areas, where the exhaust fumes from vehicles and heating systems are strongly linked to heart attacks, strokes, cancers, asthma, and lung and mental health problems, the greatest health risk from wildfires comes from microscopic particles – 2.5 microns in size, known as PM 2.5 – of unburned carbon that penetrate into the deepest part of the lungs, and so cause the most serious health problems. Over time, this affects the cardiovascular and immune systems, and the younger someone is, the more likely their breathing or physical development will be affected. One study has estimated that wildfire smoke leads to 339,000 premature deaths per year; another as many as 500,000 in a drought year.[10] Several suggest that wildfire smoke is more dangerous than the air pollution found in cities. In Australia, a single fire season may cost upwards of $2 billion, causing hundreds of smoke-related premature deaths and thousands of hospital admissions for heart attacks and breathing problems.[11] A single day breathing in the smoke of a fire as intense and widespread as the Caldor fire in the Lake Tahoe basin could be equivalent to inhaling several packets of cigarettes.

* * *

To see how smoke from global-scale fires may harm human health, I travelled twice to Indonesia. As in California or Brazil, the burning season on the main islands of Sumatra, Kalimantan (Borneo) and Java usually lasts several months as farmers and landowners clear bush and trees to make way for crops. But in both 1997 and 2015, an intense El Niño event had occurred. These entirely natural phenomena see Pacific equatorial waters warming up, triggering deep droughts in some regions and heavy rainfall in others.

In 1997 a choking yellow haze had settled over a vast area of Indonesian tropical forest and by July was drifting north to Thailand, Singapore and Malaysia, sounding the health alarms there and even further afield in Vietnam and Laos. Hooking up with forest investigator Chip Barber, we took motorised canoes from the city of Palangkaraya to follow the fires and palls of smoke hundreds of kilometres deep into the great peatlands in the heart of Borneo. Peat fires seldom burned but because the peatlands had been drained to create land for oil palm and pulp paper plantations, they were strongly suspected by environmentalists of being the source of the fires.

Aside from the suffocating heat, the inevitable headaches and burning throats, following wildfires in equatorial Indonesia is profoundly depressing. Riverside towns and villages were wreathed in an acrid, stinking blanket of half-burned vegetation mixed with industrial pollution and car exhaust fumes. Elsewhere, the smoke from newly cleared land drifted slowly north- and eastward.

The further north we travelled, the more we found fires smouldering in the peat and passed ghostly river convoys of giant tree trunks being towed south for export and barges loaded with smaller trees to take to pulp mills. A huge network of drainage canals had been carved by excavators through the swamps, dissecting the land and drying out the deep peat deposits below, making it ready to burn before being planted with palm oil or acacia trees. We stopped at one peat fire which had been smouldering metres deep, we were told, for three years and could not be extinguished.

Just thirty years ago, central Kalimantan had been largely primary forest with small-scale Dayak farmers extracting modest numbers of logs. Into this remote place, home to tigers, elephants, rhinos, orangutans and exotic birds, had dropped an alien economic model based on the rapid felling of natural forest and the planting in its place of vast oil palm and wood fibre plantations to supply the global food and pulp and paper industries. The fires may have been triggered by El Niño and the natural drought, but the culprits were clearly the loggers who, despite protests, were driving access roads through the forest, fragmenting it and making it easier for fire to catch hold and clear land, and plantation owners who were then setting fire to what remained of the forests before planting stands of acacia or palm oil trees on a truly industrial scale.

Wealthy Indonesian elites politically close to President Suharto, but financially backed by European, US, Chinese and Japanese banks, had grabbed the land from Dayak villagers and were literally stripping and burning down the third greatest tropical forest in the world to provide industrialised countries with cheap toilet and cigarette paper, newsprint, fuel additives and low-grade vegetable oil to make everything from shampoo, toothpaste, lipstick and deodorants to chocolate and fast foods.

With the rapid destruction of the land came human rights abuses, corruption and disease. From Palangkarya to Kuala Lumpur in Malaysia nearly 1,600 kilometres to the north, the air was thick, the sun a dull red glow. Face masks were obligatory. Communities had to be evacuated and people were advised to remain indoors, but wherever we saw hospitals and health clinics, they were besieged by people with asthma, bronchitis, eye complaints and other respiratory illnesses. Officially, there had been 298,125 cases of asthma, 58,095 cases of bronchitis and 1,446,120 cases of acute respiratory infection – 1.8 million in total. The real number was almost certainly far, far more.

* * *

Months after I returned to London, I got wind of a mysterious disease which had broken out in pig farms near a town called Sungai Nipah, west of the Malaysian capital of Kuala Lumpur and 1,600 kilometres north of where we had been in Indonesia. I was intrigued. Sungai Nipah was a centre of Southeast Asian food production, and hundreds of thousands of pigs were being farmed in concrete pens set among extensive commercial mango and durian fruit orchards. At the same time as the pigs were dying, pig workers were being struck down by unexplained seizures and fevers. One moment someone could be healthy, it was said, but within the hour they could neither walk nor talk and their brains had swelled up.

The immediate medical response, backed by the government wanting to reassure people, was that this was a common swine fever and a nasty but treatable Japanese encephalitis viral infection in humans spread by mosquitoes. This did not make much sense because the farmers affected were mostly ethnic Chinese and not the local Malay Muslim villagers who did not handle pigs, suggesting that the virus was transmitted by direct contact with pigs rather than mosquitoes. Nevertheless, the authorities started intensively spraying the vegetation in the villages and around the pig farms to get rid of the mosquitoes and vaccines were rushed from Japan. None of this stopped the epidemic spreading first to other pig-producing areas of Malaysia and then to a slaughterhouse in Singapore where many Malaysian pigs were sent. It was only after 1.1 million pigs had been culled and the pig industry had been ruined that the disease subsided, by which time 283 people had been infected and 109 had died.[12]

The disease was nearly as lethal as Ebola and it was only thanks to the instinct and quick reactions of a trainee virologist named Kaw Bing Chua that a global pandemic was averted. A frustrated medical doctor, Chua had been retraining as a virologist at the University of Malaysia where, while working on the blood specimens from affected pig farmers late on a Sunday night in October 1999, his UV microscope picked up what looked to him like a new paramyxovirus – a class of virus related to mumps and other respiratory diseases. He immediately called his department head at home and asked him to come quickly to the laboratory. The professor, however, was unmoved, took one look and declared it to be a contaminated slide. He told Chua to ignore it.

'I was stunned and could not believe my ears. I just could not describe my disappointment but would not dare to challenge him,' he declared years later at a university reunion in a Kuala Lumpur hotel.[13]

But Chua did not give up. Worried by his inexperience and fearful that he was possibly handling a deadly pathogen for which there was no treatment but which had already escaped into the environment and killed hundreds of people, he ignored his boss's order, isolated the virus and put it on a slide. Within twenty-four hours he had pulled strings to obtain an American visa, booked himself on a flight to Atlanta, Georgia, and rushed it to the CDC, one of the very few places in the world able to analyse a new virus. After an agonising delay when a machine did not work, it was confirmed as a new pathogen.

'I could sense it was something new and deadly,' he said. 'A sense of great fear overwhelmed me. My God! It was truly a paramyxovirus. To my limited knowledge then, all paramyxoviruses known to me spread by close contact and droplet. No wonder all the Japanese encephalitis control measures intensively carried out by the Ministry of Health failed. I really felt very sorry for the poor pig farmers and workers who were given the Japanese encephalitis vaccines, told they were protected and sent back to the farms and became infected.'[14]

It took a team of ecologists, wildlife experts, epidemiologists, vets and virologists several more years to piece together just how the disease had reached the Malaysian pig farms and to demonstrate how ecological disruption in one country could trigger a lethal disease thousands of kilometres away. Funded by a $1.4 million grant from the US National Institutes of Health, US, Australian and other scientists showed that the virus had probably been carried naturally in certain species of flying fox or horseshoe bat, which usually forage on flowering trees deep in tropical forests, but which had been forced by the smoke and flames from the Kalimantan fires to seek new food sources. Smoke had blocked the sunlight, reducing the trees' ability to flower and bear fruit, and the bats had flown off, settling on the highly productive Malaysian orchards that had been cut out of the original forests and were well fertilised with pig manure.

Pig farmers in Malaysia testified how the bats had indeed roosted above their concrete enclosures in Sungai Nipah the same year the outbreak started, and satellite tracking of the smoke plumes from the fires confirmed how the bats' habitats in Borneo were being degraded, possibly leading to their flight north to find new feeding grounds.

So what had happened? Either the fruit-loving bats had contaminated the pigs directly with virus-laden urine and faeces, or, more likely, they had dropped half-eaten fruit into the concrete pig enclosures below the trees where they were roosting. The pigs had then eaten the disease-carrying fruit and, being genetically close to humans, had amplified the potency of the virus and passed it to humans.

The theory that the smoke-filled Indonesian forests and plantations could be the source of a potential pandemic in Malaysia was stunning because it strongly suggested that complex human changes to the environment could be driving the emergence of dangerous new diseases, and that degradation of habitat in one place can set off a chain of unanticipated ecological consequences elsewhere, which could have far-reaching effects on humans and other species. The discovery of Nipah was the inspiration behind Stephen Soderbergh's 2011 Hollywood thriller *Contagion*, which tried to show how the world would react to the catastrophic escape of a deadly virus.

Nipah kills around 70 per cent of the people it infects and outbreaks occur regularly in Bangladesh and India. So far, more than 700 people have died from it and the WHO has identified it as one of eight viruses with the potential to cause a global public health emergency.[15]

*   *   *

Ten years after the link was made between smoke from forest fires and Nipah, I travelled with a Greenpeace expedition to Riau province in Sumatra, one of the most heavily logged provinces in Indonesia. There had been another deep drought in 2015 and, once again, vast areas of equatorial forest were burning. Smoke from thousands of fires was drifting from some of the world's deepest peat deposits northwards to Malaysia, Singapore, Thailand and beyond.

But instead of travelling slowly by canoe, as I had done in 1997, now it was possible to see the damage being done by global agribusiness and the pulp and paper industries from a small plane. For hour after hour we flew low over an industrial landscape of regimented palm and acacia plantations through a haze of blue smoke from fires on newly cleared land. Cross-referencing with GPS mapping and landownership maps, it was clear that the fires had mostly been started on land owned by large paper mills, and that the clearing and draining of peatlands for agribusiness had resulted in more fires than ever before.

Official figures showed that the rate of natural forest loss between 1990 and 2005 was around 1.87 million hectares per year. Now, the World Bank declared it was both a health and an environmental disaster, with more than 2.6 million hectares of forest, peat and other land burning out of control across Indonesia.[16]

It was, said Yuyun Indradi, a forest campaigner with Greenpeace Southeast Asia in Jakarta, the 'fastest, most comprehensive transformation of an entire landscape that has ever taken place anywhere in the world', including the Amazon. 'If it continues at this rate all that will be left in twenty years is a few fragmented areas of natural forest surrounded by huge man-made plantations.

There will be increased floods, fires, disease and droughts but no animals,' he said.[17]

As the number of wildfires have increased worldwide, so has the research into their health impacts. According to data from the Indonesian Health Ministry, more than 120,000 people sought medical help in 2015 because of the haze and smoke. Later Harvard and Columbia University studies suggested there had been 91,000 premature deaths.[18]

In places the haze was too thick to see through and was blanketing cities for weeks. A team led by Martin Wooster of King's College London, working with the Indonesia-based Center for International Forestry Research, tested the air pollution in Palangkaraya. It was, they said in their report, 'perhaps the worst sustained air quality ever recorded worldwide',[19] with PM10 concentrations often over 4,000µg per cubic metre for three or more weeks – far more than Beijing on one of its worst days and forty times worse than the WHO recommended level. Schools were closed for weeks, crops failed for lack of sunlight and wildlife was dying.[20] Fires in peatlands drained for plantations are a major contributor to the deadly haze that afflicts the region, smouldering for days or weeks underground in conditions which release three to six times more smoke particulates than fires elsewhere.[21]

I went to see Abetnego Tarigan, then director of WALHI, Indonesia's largest environment group. There was no doubt, he said that the smoke was creating disease as well as human rights abuses and social chaos. The legacy of deforestation was conflict, increased poverty, migration to cities, the erosion of habitat for animals, and diseases like malaria and diarrhoea.

US and European researchers followed up with major studies. Seema Jayachandran from Northwest University in Washington State used Indonesian census figures to calculate that air pollution at that time had led to more than 15,600 child and infant deaths.[22] It had been a health catastrophe.

It devastated lives. Mursyi Ali, from the village of Kuala Cenaku in the province of Riau, had spent ten years fighting oil plantation companies, which were awarded a giant concession. 'We used to have all we wanted. That all went when the companies came. Everything that we depended on went. We get new diseases. We have malaria which we only seldom had before. Our children have diarrhoea. We are all poorer now. This is life or death,' he told me.[23]

As the trees come down, so other physical processes start. Without roots to hold the soil together the land becomes more likely to be washed or blown away, and diseases emerge.

5

THE HARMED LAND

I was picked up by Mustabayev Najmedin, the mayor of Aralsk, and together with Josef, a local doctor, we drove due south on the dead-flat bed of the Aral Sea in Kazakhstan. The tyres of the battered, twenty-year-old VW Passat cut deep ruts in the salt-crusted surface and a hot, stinging wind billowed dust behind us.

Our destination was the *Alexei Leonov*, an old trawler named after the first man to have walked in space. More than a thousand tonnes of steel had been brought in pieces by train and assembled to make the boat on a slipway of the lake in the early 1970s. In those days, the Aral Sea was one of the richest fisheries on earth, famous for its bream, barbel and sturgeon. Vladimir Ulyanov (aka Lenin) had in 1921 personally asked the Aral fishers to set aside some of their catch for 'the old men and women bloated by starvation' in the great Russian famine of that year, which may have killed as many as 5 million people. They had at once responded by sending fourteen box cars full of fish to Moscow. The state of the fish after the long journey and who ate them is not recorded.

Today, thanks to a Soviet obsession with industrial-scale cotton farming and the abuse of chemicals, most of the Aral Sea is a desolate, windswept, toxic plain and the scene of one of the twentieth century's greatest man-made ecological and medical disasters. The *Alexei Leonov* was sixty kilometres away, stranded in the desert sands, and what had been the fourth largest lake in the world – surpassed only by the Caspian Sea and Lakes Superior and Victoria – was now, relatively speaking, a puddle.

It was a terrifying lesson in how disease and poverty follows human degradation of the environment. Beginning in about 1960, the great Amudarya and Syrdarya rivers and their tributaries, which flowed thousands of kilometres off the Pamir mountains in Kyrgyzstan and central Asia into the inland Aral Sea, had been diverted by Soviet premier Nikita Khrushchev's engineers to irrigate cotton and rice on an industrial scale. Hundreds of kilometres of channels and reservoirs had been dug, but while the cotton grew and the surrounding steppes bloomed, the lake died, with catastrophic effects on human health.

As the sea dried up, the natural salts and synthetic chemicals that had washed down in vast quantities from cotton and rice fields in neighbouring Uzbekistan and Kazakhstan were exposed and whipped up by the wind. The regional climate changed and the bone-dry contaminated soils were dispersed in fearsome toxic dust storms, which poisoned crops and people as they drifted hundreds of kilometres around. By some estimates more than 40 million tons of soil was blown away every year and great numbers of people who lived close to the doomed sea suffered respiratory, heart and lung problems.

The *Alexei Leonov* emerged from the dust after forty-five minutes. Raided for its metal, and abandoned with a sister ship many kilometres from the old shoreline, it lay deep in the sand-encrusted former lake bed, sheltering a family of camels and the occasional wild horse. 'The sea here was forty-four metres deep,' Najmedin told me. He had been born in 1950 in Karajalan, once a pretty Aral lakeside fishing village that was now fifty kilometres from the sea. 'We used to swim there. Dad was a fisherman. I remember going out in the boats as a family. In the holidays I caught sturgeon, carp, barbel and roach.'[1]

Dressed formally in a black coat and red hat, with fine moustaches and a mouthful of gold teeth, he was almost in tears as he recounted what had been lost, spitting his anger at the Moscow planners and scientists who had knowingly authorised the death of this sea and the slow death of a prosperous people.

> An ecological and health disaster was taking place under our eyes. There was no work, nothing. When the sea was there we were prosperous. When the sea left us, life was sad. We had neither sea nor fish. They [the Soviet leaders] took the water, they took the land, and they left us a desert. They never returned it. The climate has changed. This is man-made climate change. In winter it is colder, in summer it is hotter. Once the town was famous for its fish, now camels live here. There used to be 16,500 people fishing, we caught 6,000 tonnes of fish a year. Now we breed cows and sheep.[2]

His colleague, a doctor, took up the story.

> There are far more illnesses, over a vast area now. Our health deteriorated with the pollution that came with the winds; we had no work and many children died. In the past we had good health. Then came lung diseases, TB, heart, brain problems, cancers. People are born with disabilities. The salt and toxic dust storms, the pesticides and fertilisers made it hard to breathe. People left the town and the winters became colder and longer. Many infants died.[3]

Nalibayev Madelkhan, the director of Aralsk's small but proudly presented museum, showed us pictures of life in the 1960s. 'In the past, the sandy winds would come once or twice a month, now they occur almost daily. When the wind blew the leaves of the trees went white. There was no water for our trees. We were in despair. Nature was abused, people were abused. Our museum is dedicated to water. Water is the blood that can give life to everything. Water is our life,' he said.

We travelled from what would have been lakeside community to community, all now shrunk in size, their people fiercely proud of their resilience and the past. Resentment still ran deep: 'The

Soviet Union knew what would happen. They told people that they would bring water from Siberia to replace the Aral Sea but they never did. They were going to turn the rivers of Siberia south to grow cotton. We knew they were crazy!' said one man.[4]

But now there was hope. Thanks to help from South Korea and the World Bank, a dam had been built to hold back one of the greatly diminished rivers, returning a lake to one small part of the Aral Sea. Water levels had risen and the pike perch and carp had returned in numbers big enough to support a small fish factory. The industry may never fully recover, but it is a start. If the money is found, Aralsk may one day be only five kilometres from its sea.

* * *

Forty kilometres from Aralsk, across the desert sands in neighbouring Uzbekistan, is Vozrozhdeniya, or 'Rebirth' Island, also home to a vibrant fishing village fringed by fish-filled turquoise lagoons in the 1950s, but selected in that decade, because of its isolation, to be the site of the Soviet Union's most secret biological weapons testing research station.

It was no longer an island because sea levels had fallen, and the only traces of the thousand scientists who had lived and worked here were the abandoned, now-crumbling concrete block houses and laboratories. Here the brightest and best young Soviet biologists had used monkeys, horses, sheep and cattle to conduct great open-air experiments on anthrax, smallpox, bubonic plague and rare diseases like Q-fever, tularaemia, botulinum and Venezuelan equine encephalitis.

Vozrozhdeniya, truly in no-man's-land, was still remote, chilling and diseased. It was said to be one of the most cursed places on earth, full of dark secrets and mysteries. Stories abound of people who had died of plague and smallpox there, of boats that had strayed too close and been infected with unidentifiable diseases, of strange fish-kills, flocks of sheep losing all their wool and animals dropping dead in the brown hazes of poison that sometimes descended on it.

Here, apparently, there had been phantom military patrols, and thousands of cattle poisoned by anthrax had been buried. In May 1988 it was said that half a million saiga antelope mysteriously died in just one hour on the steppes just north of the Aral Sea. Some of the stories are explicable. The Baikonur space station is close by and it is just possible that fuel was jettisoned from rockets onto herds; equally it is known that plague is endemic in the region.

Only a very few people have been there in fifty years. One was Oxford academic geographer and adventurer Nick Middleton, who persuaded some Kazakh former fishermen – now scavengers – to take him there.[5] Middleton had taken advice from a British military expert in bioterrorism, who had told him the golden rule in places like this was not to touch anything. He had been scared stiff but came away with a haunting film.[6]

'Researchers at Rebirth Island,' he says, 'used to joke that the condemned monkeys were the luckiest inhabitants of the Soviet Union because they lived on fresh fruit. Bananas, oranges and apples were rare delicacies for most human residents of the Soviet Union, but a test animal had to remain in prime condition right up to its last breath. The cream of Soviet science, those who conducted the atmospheric trials, lived on hunks of bread and fatty sausage.'[7]

I knew that in 1999 US scientists had been sent there to clean it up, so I asked Mustabayev Najmedin if we could go there. 'No,' he said flatly in Kazakh. Besides, there was a dust storm with heavy, yellowish-tinged clouds brewing on the eastern horizon. 'Don't breathe if it hits us,' he said as we raced back to Aralsk.

* * *

What has happened to the Aral is happening all over the world and tomorrow's pandemics and major disease outbreaks could well emerge from places where land is being degraded and inland seas like the Aral are drying up. In modern times, the waters of many of the world's great lakes have been disastrously polluted and drained. Dams, irrigation projects, river diversions, the planting of inappropriate thirsty crops and the heavy use of pesticides and evaporation have changed the regional climates and badly affected people's health.

Lake Urmia in Iran, until recently the largest salt lake in the Middle East and known for its flamingoes and therapeutic mud, is now, like the Aral Sea, a fraction of the size it was fifty years ago, with nearby human populations suffering skin and heart diseases. Lakes Poopo in Bolivia, Chad in Niger and Tai in China, among others, are all shrinking fast and ecologically damaged. The result is invariably air pollution, with people suffering asthma attacks, chronic breathing and lung problems, and cardiovascular and heart diseases.

The Salton Sea, created by irrigation projects in the early twentieth century, is the US equivalent of the Aral Sea. California's largest lake is shrinking fast as water that once came to it from the Colorado river is diverted to the coast. A popular, prosperous holiday resort in the 1960s, hosting the likes of Frank Sinatra, Bing Crosby and the Beach Boys, it is now semi-deserted and ghostly, and the source of some of California's worst air pollution. The natural salts of the lake-bed sediments mix with fertilisers and pesticides from surrounding intensive farmlands and the frequent winds shower nearby communities with clouds of toxic dust. One in three people in some places suffers from asthma, bronchitis is common and many residents complain about coughing, wheezing and shortness of breath.

Just as the soils of the Fertile Crescent have been blown away since Neolithic times, so land is being blown away today. From Burkina Faso to Bihar in India and from Kansas to Kazakhstan, soil is being trashed, contaminated and stripped not out of ignorance but out of innumerable acts of wilful mismanagement and desperation for water to grow food. Those few critical centimetres closest to the surface, which contain most of the beneficial microbes and give life, are simply being washed or blown away. With the soil go the insects, fungi and microbes, and all the organic matter that provides what is needed for human health.

I spoke to soil scientist Stephan Mantel, head of the World Soil Museum in Amsterdam, who has worked around the world to try to stop soils being blown away or becoming too salty to grow food.

> Soils erode and build naturally, but very slowly. It can take a thousand years to produce a centimetre of soil, but just a few years to destroy it. In dry lands, especially, they are being lost at phenomenal rates, just as happened in the Midwest in the Dust Bowl era.
>
> I have seen half a metre of soil being lost in a very few years in places like Borneo and China. Traditional societies learned to survive by knowing how to keep in balance with nature; it is when environmental conditions change, or population increase adds to pressure on farms to produce, that the problems start. The deep ploughing of land, continual overgrazing of animals, large-scale irrigation schemes and the excessive use of fertilisers and pesticides which kill organisms have left vast acreages vulnerable to erosion and led to the onset of human malnutrition and disease.[8]

According to the UN, the world loses 24 billion tons of fertile soil a year and temperature increases and heavy rains associated with climate breakdown are further degrading already damaged soils. In some places, like the Loess Plateau of China, the highlands of Ethiopia and parts of the American Midwest, the land is beyond repair. Soil scientists are alarmed, saying that it is as if the land itself is being mined like coal or shale. The figures, which can only be approximate, are alarming. By one count, one-third of the planet's productive farmland is now severely degraded; another says around 12 million hectares a year – that's an area nearly as big as Belgium or Pennsylvania, or Malawi in Africa – are being lost annually. Add in future warming and it is predicted by the UN that crop yields could fall by 10 per cent globally,[9] and up to 50 per cent in some areas. Aside from the inevitable hunger and diseases linked to malnutrition, soil loss risks political instability and migration.

Early in 2021, researchers used satellite imagery to measure the loss of topsoil in the corn belt of the American Midwest. Edwin

Thaler and colleagues calculated that soil erosion, especially on ridges and hilltops, was so severe that about 40 million hectares had lost all their carbon-rich topsoil and that corn and soya yields had been reduced by about 6 per cent, costing farmers $3 billion a year.[10]

Modern agriculture has altered the face of the planet and the health of species more than any other human activity. It has been responsible for nearly all deforestation and soil loss, the collapse in bird populations and biodiversity, and the pollution of fresh water. The latest assessments suggest that 40 per cent of the world's land is now degraded, affecting nearly half of all humanity's health and wealth.[11]

At its most extreme, intensive farming sees the land literally blow away. In the Dust Bowl era of the 1930s, years of drought and intensive farming combined with low food prices to produce brutal dust storms and widespread illness in the Great Plains region of the US Midwest. Pioneering farmers who from the 1920s onwards had expanded on to previously untilled grasslands in the Midwest enthusiastically ploughed up the prairies to grow wheat and other crops.

Either through the belief that these good soils were inexhaustible, or greed, they ploughed the land deep, leaving the soils exposed. It was bad luck that a series of deep droughts and great storms then destroyed their work. The winds picked up the fine soil particles and vast quantities of some of the world's most fertile topsoil was blown off baked-dry, barren fields and carried hundreds of kilometres on the wind. Tens of thousands of families left with the departing soil, migrating west to camps and settlements in California.

Dust storms from the world's many drylands accelerate natural soil erosion but they do not just affect farming. Diseases, too, blow in on them, because the disturbed soil may contain seeds, spores and fungi, as well as the normally buried bacteria, viruses and pathogens and fertilisers applied to the crops.

Pathogens, it is now known, latch onto dust, and inhaling the soil and dust blown up from the Great Plains in the 1930s triggered many diseases like silicosis, bronchitis and emphysema. The state of Kansas reported a severe measles epidemic in 1931, along with abnormally high rates of infant mortality, asthma and throat and eye infections.[12] 'Dust pneumonia' is said to have killed thousands of people, clogging up lungs and causing severe allergic reactions.[13]

It reportedly took one great dust storm to reach Washington from the Great Plains in 1933 for the US government to understand the problem. Hugh Hammond Bennett, the first director of the newly formed US Soil Erosion Service, had been asked to give evidence in the Capitol even as great clouds of dust fell on the city. It helped persuade Franklin Roosevelt's new administration to put soil conservation on the political agenda for the first time. Hammond went on to be known as 'the father of soil conservation', famously saying: 'Americans have been the greatest destroyers of land of any race or people, barbaric or civilized,' adding: 'What [is] happening is sinister, a symptom of our stupendous ignorance.'[14]

Today the science is better, and drought warning systems are more certain, but another prolonged drought on the same scale as those which led to the Dust Bowl would have similar results and, given climate change, is quite likely. Improved irrigation, reservoirs and groundwater can also stave off disaster for a while, but rivers like the Colorado are already overdrawn and many aquifers are nearing depletion.

If anything, dust storms and their diseases are worsening. Ninety years after the Dust Bowl, storms exacerbated by bad farming practices are on the rise throughout the world, carrying disease from farmland to city and from continent to continent. In the American Southwest, where the climate is steadily drying, they have become so frequent in the past decades that some soil scientists fear there could be a return to the Dust Bowl era. One study, conducted in 2017, suggested there have been 2,260 dust 'events' between 1988 and 2011.[15] On average, there were approximately twenty dust storms a year recorded in the 1990s, and forty-eight a year in the 2000s – an increase of 240 per cent in two decades.

* * *

It is not just the American Midwest that is suffering from the diseases carried in the wind. Nick Middleton, one of the few men ever to have explored Vorozgnaya Island, has documented similar ecological catastrophes as farmers expanded wheat-growing into the semi-arid Argentine Pampas grasslands in the 1930s and '40s, and when Khrushchev, himself a farmer, expanded Soviet farming into the 'virgin lands' of western Siberia and northern Kazakhstan in the 1950s.[16] In both cases, tens of millions of hectares of fertile grassland were ploughed up, releasing billions of tonnes of topsoil. Today the Pampas has turned to growing soya and is in danger of losing what is left of its fertility.[17]

Now it is the turn of China, Mongolia and the Middle Eastern countries to lose their land and succumb to new diseases. Great dust storms have been recorded in these regions for centuries but growing human populations and the heavy overgrazing of animals, deforestation and the overcultivation of crops have made such storms both more frequent and larger. Vast areas of Iraq and Iran now suffer immense dust storms every year, shrouding cities and crops in a fine red dust. Made worse by climate change and droughts, as well as by the building of dams which prevent water from reaching wetlands, they bring respiratory diseases, hepatitis and cholera.

In Inner Mongolia hundreds of square kilometres of man-made desert are being created every year.[18] There, the number of people has quadrupled since 1960, while the livestock population has ballooned from 10 million in 1960 to more than 60 million today and the number of dust storms has increased sixfold. The government has invested in massive tree-planting schemes, but much of the land is barren.[19]

Showing that the wind carries individual viruses, bacteria and other pathogens over vast distances is difficult. There is much circumstantial evidence that the mysterious Kawasaki disease, which causes heart attacks in children and has been found in Hawaii and San Diego, is linked to dust storms blowing from the Gobi Desert, and in Chile to dust storms from the Atacama Desert.[20] Equally, coccidioidomycosis, or valley fever, often appears in the increasingly arid Southwest of the US after dust storms carried on the hot, dry Santa Ana winds. In 2014, 5,624 cases were diagnosed, but this increased to 10,359 by 2019. The disease, which is caused by the spores of a family of fungi found mainly in soils of the Southwest, appears to be localised. Two-thirds of all cases occur in a 'corridor' that runs through the Southwest, Mexico and Central America, and on into Brazil, Bolivia, Paraguay and Argentina.

Dust spares no one. Sinus problems, asthma, migraines, eye irritation and chest pains are not often associated with life on Caribbean islands but have all been linked to the billions of tons of sand and soil blown from West Africa and the Sahara Desert over the Atlantic in massive dust storms.[21]

* * *

Somewhere between Tamassoko and Silmiogou in eastern Burkina Faso I started shivering; soon I developed a fever and within a few hours I was sneezing, coughing and aching. Photographer Mark Edwards and I had been bumping around in old cars with groups of farmers and NGOs, inspecting waterholes and seeing how planting trees and saving water could improve the lives of people trying to farm degraded, baking land. Years of overgrazing cattle, tree felling and ploughing up fragile soils had left an arid, denuded landscape, and bare and crusted soils scattered with thorn bushes.

Our hosts were worried enough to ask a local doctor to check me out. Mohamed, a Mossi tribesman, came from a long line of traditional African healers but he had also trained in Western medicine in France. He diagnosed my problem quickly as a short-lived, flu-like bacterial illness and gave me some antibiotics. Whatever it was that I had caught, he said, was probably caused by the wind.

The wind? It was the start of the Saharan winter and the notorious, regular-as-clockwork Harmattan was starting to gust in from the north and east, sometimes dimming the sun and filling the hot air with pollen grains, sand and dust. One thousand kilometres south on the West African coast, this same wind used to be known as the 'the doctor' because of its invigorating dryness compared with humid tropical air. Up here on the Sahelian savannah, it was an 'ill wind', often bringing colds and far worse.

Mohamed said he was seeing many more respiratory infections like asthma, coughs, sore throats, flu and pneumonia these days because there was more soil and dust in the air. The soil in this part of Burkina Faso was literally being blown away, he said, because so many trees and bushes had been cut down in the past thirty years to make way for farming and so many chemicals were being put on the land that it was breaking up.

What he had feared, he told me as he left, was meningitis. This disease occurs everywhere in the world, but by far the highest incidence is in the 'meningitis belt', a strip of countries stretching south of the Sahara from Senegal in the west to Ethiopia in the east and including Burkina Faso, northern Ghana, Nigeria and Niger. There were many cases every year, but once a decade or so there was a devastating meningitis epidemic affecting tens of thousands of people. Burkina Faso was a disease hotspot and this was one of those years. 'You are lucky,' he said as he left on a motorbike. 'It can act fast. Sometimes people go to sleep and never wake up.'

There are bacterial, viral, parasitic and fungal forms of meningitis and you really do not want to get any of them. Some, like the bacterial version, known as meningococcal meningitis, are carried on the wind and are highly contagious. This kind can spread from person to person and kills nearly one in ten of its victims. In all cases the protective membranes around the brain and neck swell painfully, leading to terrible headaches, high fevers, vomiting and extreme stiffness. The disease used to be rare but probably became endemic in the 1980s when a succession of epidemics hit hard.

In meningitis in the Sahel, as in so many other diseases, man's hand was everywhere. Global heating here is having a more severe effect than in almost any other region of Africa, and despite small-scale efforts to hold the sand back, the semi-arid land has become increasingly desert-like and degraded since the 1940s. The soils that naturally contain the bacteria or spores that lead to the disease are more easily whipped up and can be spread further on the winds.

Once sporadic and contained to the region, meningitis is now a global disease. There are vaccines, but epidemics pop up often unexpectedly, in remote refugee camps, among Haj pilgrims and even at scout jamborees.[22] Add to that increased human and cattle populations, deforestation, more disturbance of the land through ploughing and more movement of people, and all the conditions are in place for an international disaster.

Dust is now everywhere. In most ecosystems, harmful viruses, bacteria and fungi are naturally kept in check and pose little risk to human health. But in disturbed and degraded soil ecosystems, pathogens can, directly or indirectly, cause diseases in humans. Weather extremes, the overuse of land, pollution and the chemicals and antibiotics which end up there from farming operations, as well as a changing climate, make it more likely that soils will harbour disease.

* * *

It could have been the edge of the Sahara or even Death Valley, but it was actually a large orchard near Cartagena in southern Spain. On one side of a farm track the soil had broken down into fine white, lifeless sand and a landscape of rock and dying trees stretched into the distance. On the other side, kilometres of healthy trees were laden with grapefruit, lemons and oranges, while birds sang and flitted in and out of the shadows.

The line between desert and abundance in southern Spain has always been fine. In this case it was a two-and-a-half-centimetre thick black plastic pipe that dripped water pumped from a deep borehole to the base of some trees but not to others. Señor Lorenzo, who farmed 400 hectares, decided to cut off the water supply to 15,000 trees earlier this year when he was told his annual allocation of water had been heavily cut. He now farms just 200 hectares.

He tipped back his hat and mopped his brow in the scorching 42°C heat of the mid-afternoon. 'What can I do?' he asked. His reservoir was nearly empty, he had no access to more water until next year and had sacked all but two of his migrant workers, and soon he would join neighbouring fruit farmers in cutting down and burning his dead trees.

He reckoned the company that owned the farm would lose millions of euros that year. 'This is as close to a disaster as you can get,' he says. 'Everyone around here is more or less in the same situation. We have not seen anything like this before.'[23]

Alarm bells are ringing. Much of Southern Europe is now bone dry, dun-brown and baking for many months of the year. Droughts are deeper[24] and longer-lasting than ever before, heatwaves are becoming more frequent and rainfall is more torrential.[25] Southern Spain, large parts of Portugal, Italy and France and great areas in the east of the Mediterranean are all slowly desertifying, their soils drying up and blowing away. Soil erosion, says the EU, now affects a quarter of all Europe's agricultural farmland.

Patricio García-Fayos, the bearded head of the Desertification Research Centre (CIDE) in Valencia, immediately made the link between droughts, soil degradation, plant diseases and desertification:

When temperatures increase, just like people sweat more, plants transpire more, so water evaporates from soil and vegetation. These conditions weaken the plants, which makes them more vulnerable to plagues like xylella [a bacterial disease]. Even if vegetation doesn't get hit with plagues, it gets drier and more susceptible to fires. This increases the frequency and intensity of forest fires. Then, after fires, more opportunistic, dryer plants move into the area because the climatic conditions are harsher than normal. It's a vicious circle.[26]

Drylands and semi-arid countries cover 40 per cent of the world's terrestrial surface and all are now vulnerable to drying out, he said. Some are particularly at risk. Drought, overgrazing, fire and deforestation have exposed nearly 40 million hectares of soil in Iran. Over-farming and droughts in Sudan have shifted the boundary between desert and semi-desert almost 200 kilometres southward in less than a hundred years.[27]

Soil erosion is not a high priority among governments and farmers because it usually occurs so slowly that its cumulative effects take decades to become apparent, said David Pimentel, professor of agricultural sciences at Cornell University in an interview not long before he died in 2019. 'The removal of one millimetre of soil is so small that it goes undetected. But over a twenty-five-year period the loss would be twenty-five millimetres, which would take about five hundred years to replace by natural processes.'

Soil erosion in most developing countries leads in a straight line to reduced crop yields, then to poverty and migration, and finally to disease. A 50 per cent reduction in soil organic matter has been found to reduce corn yields by 25 per cent. Countries are losing soil at different rates. The US, which just avoided turning the Great Plains into a dust bowl in the 1930s, is still losing soil eighteen times more rapidly than it is forming it.

Deserts are now advancing from Africa to China as people and their animals put pressure on the land. In China, the Gobi is marching eastwards and is now within 240 kilometres of Beijing. Satellite images show the Bardanjilin Desert in north-central China pushing southward towards the Tengry Desert to form a single, larger desert, overlapping Inner Mongolia and Gansu provinces. To the west in Xinjiang province, two much larger deserts – the Taklamakan and the Kumtag – are also heading for a merger.

Wang Tao, a leading desert scholar and deputy director of the Chinese Cold and Arid Regions Environmental and Engineering Research Institute, reports that on average 156,000 hectares were converted to desert each year from 1950 until 1975. From 1975 to 1987 this increased to 210,000 hectares a year. But in the 1990s it jumped to 360,000 hectares annually, more than doubling in one generation. The human toll is heavy, but rarely is it carefully measured. Wang Tao estimates that 24,000 villages 'have been buried [by drifting sand], abandoned or endangered seriously by sandy desertification' affecting some 35 million people. In effect,

Chinese civilisation is retreating before the drifting sand that covers the land, forcing farmers and herders to leave. Most of this abandonment has occurred over the last two decades.[28]

While much is known or still being discovered about air and water pollution, no systematic study has ever been done of the global scale of soil contamination and the health effects it may be having. But in 2018 the UN's Food and Agriculture Organization (FAO) brought 500 soil scientists to Rome to assess the problem. One after another they reported not only increases in spills of 'legacy' pollutants like oils, pesticides and heavy metals such as lead and cadmium but an inexorable rise of what they termed 'emerging' pollutants, like antibiotic-resistant bacteria, hormone disruptors, micro- and nanoplastics, flame retardants and personal care products such as sanitiser wipes, sprays and gels.[29]

What was most alarming was the speed at which these contaminants are getting into the soil and countries' inability to regulate them. In sixty years, says Natalia Rodríguez Eugenio, a soil scientist from Italy, the pesticide industry alone has developed more than 800 active chemicals, many of which are used widely and remain active in the environment for years.[30] Contamination of soils by heavy metals and plastics is now out of control. Plastic has been found in the deepest trenches of the Pacific Ocean and on the highest mountains, as well as in rivers and farmland.

Just before the Covid-19 pandemic started, I went to Amsterdam to have my blood tested by Dutch marine toxicologist Dick Vethaak. It was known that huge amounts of plastic waste now contaminate the planet, from the summit of Everest to the deepest oceans. People, too, were known to consume the tiny particles via food and water but blood had never been tested.

It took nearly two years for the study to be published and when it was, it was dynamite. Of the twenty-two people tested, seventeen had microparticles in their blood; half contained PET plastic, which is commonly used in drinks bottles, while a third contained polystyrene, used for packaging food and other products. A quarter of the blood samples contained polyethylene, from which plastic carrier bags are made.

No one yet knows what effect contaminated food may be having on the health of humans or animals, but Qu Dongyu, director-general of the FAO, was frank. 'This thin crust of the Earth's surface, the soil, supports all terrestrial life and is essential to human health and well-being. Global soils are under great pressure.'[31]

6

LOSING THE PLOT

Just occasionally, a date, a name and even a time can be put to a final act of extinction. On the morning of 3 June 1844, three fishermen, Sigurður Ísleifsson, Ketill Ketilsson and Jón Brandsson, clambered on to the small island of Eldey, fifteen kilometres off the coast of Iceland. They had been contracted to collect specimens of a flightless, penguin-like bird that had once bred on remote north Atlantic islands in large numbers but which was becoming rarer and rarer.

The rocks were covered with guillemots and gannets but the men immediately recognised the large, hooked beaks and small wings of the bird which they called the 'garefowl' but is now known more widely as the great auk. A pair was standing together incubating a single egg and what happened next was described years later by Sigurður Ísleifsson to the English naturalist John Wolley. It summarises humankind's hastening of extinction over the past 200 years.

Jón Brandsson crept up with his arms open. The bird that Jón got went into a corner but [mine] was going to the edge of the cliff. It walked like a man ... but moved its feet quickly. [I] caught it close to the edge – a precipice many fathoms deep. Its wings lay close to the sides – not hanging out. I took

. him by the neck and he flapped his wings. He made no cry.
I strangled him.[1]

Even as Jon and Sigurður were throttling the birds, Ketill Ketilsson was literally putting the boot in, smashing the last egg with his foot and so ending a line of life that stretched back as much as 5 million years.

Extinctions do not usually happen with a heavy boot or in front of witnesses on a remote island. Mostly they go unseen and unrecorded. The final demise of the great auk had been predicted nearly sixty years before by explorer George Cartwright, who recalled the 'incredible destruction' of the bird for the sake of its feathers. 'If a stop is not soon put to that practice the whole breed will be diminished to almost nothing,' he wrote.[2]

The great auk was hunted first for its flesh by mariners and indigenous North American groups; then by collectors who sought its eggs; and lastly by the bedding industry, which wanted its feathers. In contrast, the North Island laughing owl, known for its gorgeous swooping flight and maniacal 'ho-ho-ho' laugh, was not desired by humanity. Instead, it disappeared by accident from the forests and hills of New Zealand because humans were ecologically clueless. Its relationship to other animals was delightfully uncomplicated. It ate anything. When ornithologists analysed the bones on a site where the birds were known to have roosted for many years, they found that its diet included forty-three species of native bird, three species of bat and two of frog, as well as fish, beetles, lizards and weevils, even a seal.

Its end – possibly cheered by the many species on which it so freely dined – came when nineteenth-century colonial farmers imported stoats and ferrets to kill off the rabbits that they themselves had earlier introduced for sport but which had got out of control. The last laughing owl was found dead on a roadside not far from a sheep station near Christchurch in 1914, although some ornithologists swear they heard one calling in a forest forty years later. It's conceivable, but highly unlikely, that there is a remnant bird or two somewhere in the great forests and mountains of North Island.

The great auk and the laughing owl are just two birds on an ever-lengthening roll of extinctions – along with other birds like the dodo, the passenger pigeon, the moa, the red rail, the giant elephant bird, the huia, Pallas's cormorant and hundreds of others which have disappeared in the last century and a half. They join thousands of mammals like the desert rat-kangaroo in Australia, the Saint Lucia giant rice rat and the many species of bees, beetles, dragonflies, fish, fleas, fungi, moths, spiders and wasps that have been hunted out of existence, prized as trophies or had their habitats whittled away and then destroyed by humans around the world. Some, like the great auk and the laughing owl, are remembered today mainly as exhibits in museums. Most are biological ghosts.

According to scientists at the International Union for the Conservation of Nature (IUCN), the world authority on global population trends for species, some 570 plant species and 700-odd animal species have gone extinct since 1500. The end of species is now happening a hundred times faster than the natural evolutionary rate, and it's accelerating.

But we don't actually know what has been lost, any more than we know exactly what remains. In 2020 the UN made a stab at putting easily understood headline figures on the ledger of life, trawling through 15,000 studies and peer-reviewed science papers to assess the state of the natural world.

The 500 or more scientists who worked on the awkwardly named Intergovernmental Platform on Biodiversity and Ecosystem Services (IPBES) took three years to compile the first global assessment of the state of the living world and shocked themselves and the world by concluding that life was being lost at a rate unprecedented in human history. Birds, mammals, amphibians and reptiles are all in accelerating decline, their populations getting smaller day by day. Around 1 million species out of an estimated 8 million on earth are now threatened with extinction, including 500,000 plants and animals and the same number of insects. The researchers had not expected this great silencing of the natural world so soon. Not only was there no telling which species were most likely to be made extinct first, or over what period of time, but they saw the cumulative loss as a massive, systemic failure by humanity to protect both itself and the life-forms on which it and the whole earth depends.

I spoke to the chair of the IPBES panel, Bob Watson, one of the most influential scientists in the world having led global studies on climate, drought and biodiversity, who told me:

> We're losing biodiversity at a rate that is truly unprecedented
> in human history. We are eroding nature's ability to provide
> the 'services' like clean air and fertile soil which we depend on.
> We have already lost nearly 90 per cent of the wetlands around
> the world. We've transformed the forests and grasslands, we've
> converted 75 per cent of the land that is not covered by ice.[3]

Professor Elizabeth Hadly at Stanford, who has spent forty years studying the links between ecology and evolution, put it into context:

> What's different is that [extinction] is happening
> simultaneously in the Amazon, in Africa, in the Arctic.
> It's happening not at one place and not with one group of
> organisms but with all biodiversity everywhere on the planet.
> Driving around, we don't have moths, butterflies, bees or all
> sorts of insects on our windshield anymore and that is scary
> because they form the food chain for hundreds of thousands of
> other species and they are extremely important for pollination.[4]

* * *

But would it really matter if there were 5, 10 or 20 per cent fewer animals, half as many plants or insects? Is it really important for human health that insects are in steep decline, or that we are losing butterfly, mammal and bird species? Surely extinction and the rise and decline of species are natural processes; and is it not the case that 95 per cent or more of all the millions of life-forms that have ever lived on earth have disappeared at some time or other and new species are continually evolving? Indeed, don't the fossil records suggest that there have been at least five previous mass extinctions and many smaller ones, all caused by massive natural shifts in the climate, sea-level rise, habitat loss and temperature change?

The head of the Biodiversity Institute in the Zoology Department at the University of Oxford, Katherine Willis, argues that it is not the numbers that are going extinct or declining but the speed at which it takes place that is important. 'Extinction is a natural process. Things come, they grow, their populations get huge and then they decline. But it's the rate of extinction that's the problem. When you look at previous groups in the fossil records, then it's over millions of years that they go extinct. Here we're looking at tens of years. All groups in the natural world are in decline, which means their populations are getting smaller, day by day,' writes Willis. 'What we now know about the natural world is that everything is joined up from a single pond to a whole tropical rainforest. All biodiversity is interlocked on a global scale and all parts of that system are required to make it function.'[5] What matters more than the fate of individual animals – and is critical for survival and our own health as a species – is the speed at which life is disappearing and the accumulating loss of genetic variety.[6]

Until recently it was hoped that the rate at which new species were evolving could keep pace with the extinctions. Working from fossil records, biologists at the IUCN calculate that extinction rates are now 100–1,000 times higher today than the background evolutionary rate and is accelerating.[7] Many species, they say, are going from relative abundance to absolute extinction in hundreds of years, even decades, rather than in thousands of years. For the first time since the end of the dinosaurs nearly 55 million years ago, humans are driving animals and plants to extinction faster than new species can evolve. Already one in four of all plant and animal groups are now threatened to some extent, along with two in five amphibian species and one in three reef-forming corals. By any measure it is an unprecedented ecological crisis.

One reason often given for humans to try to protect rare plants is naked self-interest. Most of the medicines and drugs ever developed and the biomedical research ever conducted rely on plants, animals and microbes. There are possibly 35,000 plants already known to be of some medicinal use, and there are hundreds of thousands more whose properties are not yet known. When we lose rainforests, coral reefs, savannas and mangrove swamps to farming, dams and suburbs, we may well be losing the chance of discovering the blockbuster drug needed to cure the next pandemic.

The natural world has always been the source of medicinal cures and drugs. The opium poppy gave the world codeine and morphine painkillers; quinine, used for malaria, is from the *Cinchona calisaya* tree from South America; digitalis, or foxglove, is used for heart failure; ergotamine extracted from rye treats migraines, and willow bark, or salicylates, gave us aspirin. Many of the most trusted antibiotics – like myriocin, streptomycin and erythromycin – are derived from soil fungi. Another fungus, *Isaria sinclairii*, is used to treat conditions such as multiple sclerosis.

But as human populations grow rapidly, the demand for both traditional and mainstream Western drugs is soaring, with the result that many of the world's most important medicinal plant species are being over-harvested. One survey in 2016 by botanists at the world's leading botanic gardens found trees being stripped of their bark, the roots of plants dug up and traditional controls being widely ignored. They identified 400 medicinal plants that are being over-harvested to the point of extinction and 10,000 more which are threatened.[8]

Paclitaxel, one of the world's most important cancer drugs, is derived from the bark of several species of yew, but over-harvesting in Afghanistan, India and Nepal has decimated wild yew populations across the world, with 80 per cent of the trees in China's Yunnan province, once famous for its yew forests, destroyed within a three-year period, according to the report. The tree has had to be put on the red, or endangered, list of plants.[9] The African cherry tree (*Prunus africana*) is prized by drug companies to combat malaria, kidney and prostate disorders, but the $200 million trade in its bark leaves the species' existence hanging by a thread. Hoodia, a cactus-like succulent plant native to the Kalahari Desert and used by the bushmen of Namibia to stave off hunger, is also threatened, along with autumn crocus, a natural treatment for gout and linked to helping fight leukaemia.[10]

Just as Europeans, and later North Americans, made a business of importing exotic plants like peppers, sugar, cotton, potatoes and tobacco from their colonies, so 'bio-prospecting', or the hunt for novel chemical compounds in plants to be used for drugs, is accelerating. This multi-billion-dollar-a-year business sees grants awarded to drug and food companies to scour the world for plants used especially by traditional healers in the world's indigenous groups.

Possibly one in ten of the world's 60,000 known tree species are thought to have medicinal or aromatic use and one in four of all modern pharmaceuticals are ultimately derived from rainforest plants,[11] yet fewer than one in 100 tropical plants have even been analysed for medical purposes.

The race is now on to commercialise nature, and it is being led by governments and the global drug giants. The US National Cancer Institute has reportedly collected and genetically screened over 50,000 plant and animal samples from plants and microorganisms in thirty countries.[12] The US Army holds gene patents on dozens of tropical disease treatments, including a Pacific plant called mamala (*Homalanthus acuminatus*), used in Samoa as a medicine, and microorganisms that could be used in biological warfare. Corporations have tried, unsuccessfully, to gain exclusive access to the genetic material of every plant in botanically rich countries in Latin America.

* * *

On a planetary scale there is no debate about the need to stem the tide of extinctions to protect human health. The abundance and infinite variety of life clearly determines the global climate, the regional weather and the ability of humans and other life-forms to grow food and survive. What is much less appreciated is that biodiversity is the source of all health, not only protecting humans from natural disasters like floods and storms; but cleaning water and regenerating the soils which provide food and drink. As the 2004 Asian tsunami showed, the devastating floods hit hardest where the mangrove forests on the shorelines had been removed to provide sandy beaches for tourist developments.

And, at the most intimate level, the human microbiota – those vast, infinitely diverse and barely understood communities of microbes which live symbiotically in our guts, skin and respiratory tracts – all are known to contribute to our nutrition, regulate our immune system and prevent infections.

But there is a fierce debate over whether the global loss of biodiversity that the world is seeing now increases or decreases the risk of specific disease and pandemics. One argument goes that any animal that threatens to spill disease over to humans should be killed – a practice widely used by governments to control the spread of bird and swine flus. When Covid-19 emerged, there were bat-killing sprees in Rwanda, Cuba, Indonesia, Nepal, Peru and elsewhere to destroy bat roosts in case the disease was passed on. One company, Oxitec, has already released in more than fifteen countries more than 1 billion male mosquitoes genetically engineered to carry a protein that will kill off any female offspring before they reach mature biting age on the basis that this could reduce the spread of diseases like dengue, malaria and schistosomiasis. The long-term effects are not known.[13]

Killing wildlife to protect humans misses the point about the need for biodiversity. Mosquitoes are important pollinators and a food source for birds, fish and frogs; bats provide invaluable pest control and pollination services. Aside from being next to impossible because there are so many species, if we were to destroy bats' roosts or eradicate mosquitoes, the consequences up and down the food chain are uncertain.

Not only might their ecological niches be filled by even more dangerous species, but disease ecologists warn that it runs the risk of concentrating pathogens in the remaining animal populations, so replicating the disastrous behaviour that led to viruses jumping species in the first place. Mark Jones, a vet working with the Born Free Foundation in Horsham, UK, is clear: 'Extinction of bat roosts won't do anything to reduce the risk of another human pandemic. We can't go around trying to eliminate the risk by exterminating animals in the wild.'[14]

'There are many ways to remove pieces of the puzzle. The most obvious way is to kill something, and we do a lot of that. We tend to think that we're somehow outside of that system, but we are part of it and we are totally reliant upon it. We're in a big, very fast-driving vehicle and there is a giant wall ahead of us. The question is, can we stop in time? We have done amazing things in the past very quickly when we rally together,' says Stanford University biology professor Elizabeth Hadly.[15]

Blame for the rising number and increasing lethality of infectious diseases that humans suffer should not lie with the animals that are passing the diseases to us, but with the humans who are changing the environment and so creating the conditions for them to emerge, say ecologists. Not only are we threatening the survival of so many species, but by killing them we are increasing the risk of spillover and disease. It is this unfortunate convergence that has led to the linked environmental and health mess which we find ourselves in today.

Years of research by wildlife epidemiologist Christine Kreuder Johnson, director of the EpiCenter for Disease Dynamics at the UC Davis School of Veterinary Medicine, and other disease ecologists in the US and Australia, made a firm link in 2020 between human actions and the diseases that are emerging. In a paper which strongly suggested that the underlying cause of Covid-19 was likely to be increased human contact with wildlife, they took 142 viruses known to have been transmitted from animals to humans since 1940 and matched them to the IUCN's Red List of threatened species.[16]

Johnson told me how nearly half of all the new diseases that jumped from animals could now be traced to human action. SARS, Ebola, West Nile, Lyme, MERS and others all emerged, in effect, as a result of humans encroaching on animals' habitats. When she and her colleagues traced which animals were most likely to share pathogens with humans, they found that wild animals that have increased in abundance and adapted well to human-dominated environments shared more viruses with people. These included some rodent, bat and primate species that live among people, near our homes and around our farms and crops, making them high-risk for ongoing transmission of viruses to humans. Together they were implicated as hosts for nearly 75 per cent of all viruses. Bats alone have been linked to diseases like SARS, Nipah, Marburg and Ebola.

At the other end of the spectrum, the team looked at threatened and endangered species. These were predicted to host twice as many zoonotic viruses compared to threatened species whose populations were decreasing for other reasons.[17] Their conclusion was stark: by denuding nature, we risk more viruses spilling over from animals to humans.

* * *

Meanwhile, there is growing interest in the way that new diseases affecting humans may be linked to the erosion of biodiversity. Two remarkable biologists, Felicia Keesing from Bard College, New York, and Rick Ostfeld, based at the Cary Institute of Ecosystem Studies in Millbrook, also in New York, had spent decades studying tick-borne illnesses in the forests of the Hudson Valley in New York State and in the savannas of East Africa.

They found that when we erode biodiversity we increase the chances of diseases passing from one species to another. In an intact forest or other ecosystem, they say, the diversity of the creatures in it 'dilutes' the impact of the generally smaller creatures like rats and mice, which 'amplify' diseases like Lyme disease, West Nile virus, African and American trypanosomiasis and some forms of leishmania.[18]

This 'dilution effect' suggests that high biodiversity acts as a protection against some infectious diseases being transmitted, says Ostfeld:

When humans destroy habitat, there are definite winners and losers. The losers tend to be the bigger animals which have highly specific feeding requirements and are comparatively larger, rarer and longer-lived. The winners tend to be small and abundant, animals which lead 'fast', short lives like rats and mice, which proliferate wildly, live at super high density. These are far more likely to make us sick.

Often the best reservoirs for the pathogens that can jump to humans are these smaller-bodied species, like rats and mice and certain kinds of bats. When we have intact natural systems with high biodiversity, these species are kept in check. But when humans destroy habitat, the large predators and herbivores disappear first.[19]

'When we humans do things that erode biodiversity, we're effectively getting rid of the helpful species and favouring the nasty ones,' adds Keesing.

The 'dilution effect' has been shown as likely to apply to Lyme disease as well as West Nile virus in the US, but Ostfeld and Keesing do not claim that it applies to all species in all environments. Nevertheless, their idea is ground-breaking and gaining support. Its tentative implications for conservation and human health are potentially enormous, suggesting that money invested in conservation has a positive health benefit, too.[20] According to Keesing, 'What we're finding out is that the protection of human health is one of many major ecosystem services provided by biodiversity.'[21]

* * *

The point that humans are largely responsible for the emergence of disease was underlined in early 2020 when twenty-two of the world's leading zoologists, public health and economic experts were asked by the UN to assess whether Covid-19 and other pandemics could be linked to the way humans treat nature. They went back over all the reports that linked human disease with animal pathogens and concluded that this was the Age of Pandemics. Moreover, they said, the risk of more pandemics was increasing rapidly, with possibly five new diseases crossing the species barrier into humans from animals every year.[22]

Not only have all pandemics in recorded history had their origins in microbes carried by wildlife, they said, but science had identified only about 2,000 of the 1.7 million viruses known to exist in birds and mammals. Between 540,000 and 850,000 of these viruses could spill over to infect humans. Unless steps are taken, pandemics will emerge more often, spread faster, kill more people and do more economic damage.

The authors of the report summarised the latest understanding of the emergence of pandemics. This suggests that not only are they becoming more frequent, but that they are emerging as a direct result of human activities: the same activities – land-use change, agricultural expansion and global trade – that are also driving the loss of nature and climate change. In other words, they concluded, the forces that are destroying nature are the same ones that are creating the conditions for pandemics like Covid-19 to emerge.

They spelled the situation out. Human disruption of nature and unsustainable consumption were the twin problems. Most emerging diseases originated in nature-rich developing countries, but were being driven by demand for natural resources in wealthy countries. It made sense, but I wanted to know how far our actions were leading to the emergence of specific diseases.

NATURE IN THE HUMAN WORLD

Where I live on the wooded border of Wales and England, we do not expect to catch tropical diseases or think that the plants and animals we see on our walks will harm us. How wrong can we be? These borderlands, with their ancient forests, small rivers and mixed farms, may have repelled invading English armies for millennia, but like everywhere else they are now succumbing to successive biological invasions and global pandemics of plants, people and animals. We may live far from world cities and tropical rainforests, but we are learning that we are connected to all other life by disease.

In just the past year – aside from major outbreaks of Covid-19 in nearby care homes and meat-packing plants – there have been several strange clusters of Mpox, a nasty smallpox-like disease normally confined to remote villages in the Democratic Republic of Congo, as well as incidents of highly contagious bird and horse flu. Lyme disease, a debilitating condition caught from ticks feeding on sheep on the nearby moors, is becoming common, HIV/Aids is prevalent in the nearest town and historic diseases like TB are circulating again. And that's just within a few kilometres.[1]

In 1897 David Lloyd George, the British prime minister, called our valley 'a little bit of heaven on earth', and it has changed less than most. The banks of the river Ceiriog, which tumbles down from the wild Berwyn mountains, are now lined with Himalayan balsam, a pretty enough plant with pink orchid-like flowers which was brought to Britain from India in 1939; the red squirrels that were once common here have long given way to greys; harlequin ladybirds, which flew in from Asia ten years ago, have found an ecological niche and are now displacing native species; poultry farmers report bird flu, probably from mainland Europe; giant hogweed, an impressive but toxic plant originally from the Caucasus mountains, is just thirty kilometres away; and now *Phytophthora pluvialis*, a serious tree disease first seen in Oregon only in 2013, is said to be close.

Landscapes change continually and with the changes we must expect new diseases. The crowns of the tall ash trees across the river show unmistakable signs of die-back, a fungal disease thought to have arrived from Asia in 2006. It is only the latest in a long series of devastating tree diseases to hit Britain. Dutch elm in the 1960s was followed by a new Phytophthora disease that weakened and killed alders along riverbanks in the 1990s. Millions of larches have had to be felled and oaks, beeches and conifers are all under sustained attack from the pests, fungi and diseases that have arrived since the horticultural trade became truly global in the 1980s.

It is not only in Britain that the health of both the natural world and humans is being rapidly impacted by global invasions. From Wuhan to Wellington and Birmingham to Baltimore, exotic bugs, ants, spiders, fish, mites, moths, ticks, reptiles, birds, beetles, amphibians and other pests and insects are arriving on pallets, in cardboard boxes and in the soil of ornamental plants. Stowing away on the bottom of boats and the backs of imported pets, swimming in on warmer seas, some pose new health challenges.

Like humans, plants are beset by viruses, bacteria, fungi and parasites. As with humans, most are beneficial and very few of the many thousands of new species which make it to any country every year will live long, let alone adapt themselves to new climates and go on to breed and spread disease.

The movement of exotic bugs today goes in every direction and is unstoppable. But because they have evolved separately over millennia, they travel with unique pathogens, fungi and bacteria.

The result is that those that are able to adapt are likely to dramatically change environments and endanger human health.

* * *

Undermining human health more than any other species is a slender fly with two wings, three pairs of long legs and a very large mouth adapted over millennia to pierce the skin of any animal and suck its blood. There may be as many as 100 trillion mosquitoes, and their 3,500 or more species spread at least twenty lethal human diseases, which together are thought to infect nearly 700 million people a year.

Mosquitoes are on a roll globally, and thanks to humans, who are creating the perfect habitats for them to breed and spread, they are expanding their range further and faster than any other insect. They have been with us for millennia, breeding first in tropical swamps, wetlands and marshes, but it took nineteenth-century shipping, trade and colonialism to really expand their range. Today mosquitoes occupy just about every corner of the world except Antarctica, kill nearly 500,000 people a year and are adapting to live at higher altitudes and even underground.

Most dangerous of all the many invasive species is the Asian tiger mosquito (*Aedes albopictus*), which probably originated in the forests and wetlands of Southeast Asia but has recently adapted to exploit most human habitats. In the last thirty years, its numbers have exploded. First found in Texas in 1985,[2] today it is breeding in at least forty US states, moving rapidly towards Central and South America, and established in the Caribbean and most Mediterranean countries.[3] Almost certainly *Albopictus* is coming to a country near you.

I turned to Michael 'Doc' Weissman, chief entomologist at the Colorado Mosquito Control company in Denver, Colorado, who has been on the frontline of insect control in the state for more than thirty years. He is paid to eradicate mosquitoes, but has a barely disguised respect for *Albopictus*, alternatively calling it 'gorgeous' and 'stunning' with its dark body, silvery scales and distinctive white stripe. 'She's a beauty, but she packs a deadly punch. Most mosquitoes are vampire-like in their avoidance of the sun, waiting until after sunset to seek a blood meal; this one bites during the daytime in full sunlight,' he says.[4]

No other mosquito species has adapted so well to humans, he thinks. While most evolved to live in warm and humid swamps, in marshes and at forest edges, the tiger is a 'container breeder', meaning that its larvae thrive in small containers of water. In their native habitats, they lay their eggs in tree holes, puddles, rock pools and even coconut shells, but in the past forty years they have adapted to cooler places and moved to cities, where they breed in any small items that hold water.

Possibly they got a taste for travel and the West at the end of the Vietnam War, when millions of military tyres were returned to the US on the decks of ships. The tyres were the perfect shape for breeding, holding rainwater and preventing the larvae from drying out. The US car trade did the rest, taking the insect to most US cities and abroad. Equally, *Albopictus* may have arrived with the horticulture trade in ornamental bamboo shoots. Now it has learned to breed in rubbish bins, watering cans, gutters, flowerpots, blocked drains, even bird baths, and it can survive freezing temperatures.

Albopictus is the world's most worrisome invasive species because it relies almost entirely on humans, outcompetes other mosquito species and is able to transmit some of the world's most severe illnesses, including West Nile virus, dengue, chikungunya, Zika and yellow fever. As human populations expand, and *Albopictus* learns to adapt even better, it's almost certain to spread further. Some epidemiologists believe it is already in the UK and likely to arrive in every city in temperate regions within a few years.

* * *

Myriad species of bugs, beetles, flies and other insects directly harm humans, mostly with mild bites and stings, rashes and allergic reactions. But there is reason to think that because of changing temperatures and environments, many which were never considered a problem before are changing their populations, finding they can flourish in new places and becoming more dangerous, say Italian entomologists Giuseppe Mazza and Elena Tricarico.

These two Florentine biologists study the way invasive species affect human health. They fear not only that humans are losing the fight to stop them spreading, but that the rate of introduction of those with adverse health effects on humans is increasing, with no evidence of saturation. 'Effects on human health vary. They range from psychological effects, phobias, discomfort and nuisance to allergies, poisonings, bites, disease and death,' says Tricarico.[5]

Rather than blame arriving species and try to eradicate them with ever more powerful chemicals, they argue that we should understand that it is our own actions that encourage them to invade and change nature. And if we don't like them, rather than try to eradicate them, which is messy and usually unsuccessful, we might do better to address the conditions that enable them to migrate and spread.

Invasive species don't just affect human health directly. Indirectly, many are creating poverty and reducing human resilience by lowering crop yields, restricting access to water, reducing fish catches and weakening immune systems. I saw this first on the White Nile in Uganda, where water hyacinth (*Pontederia crassipes*) was rampant along hundreds of kilometres of river from Lake Victoria north through Uganda and into Sudan. Close to Juba, its dense and impenetrable mats were blocking dams and irrigation channels and preventing hydropower stations from working.

Near Lake Victoria, I watched tourists pose for photographs in front of its pretty flowers, unaware that this floating aquatic plant, which probably came to Africa with Belgian colonists, is a monster, able to double its spread in a few weeks. Dubbed the 'million dollar weed', the 'Bengal terror' and the 'blue devil', it is virtually out of control and a perfect habitat for malaria- and dengue-carrying mosquitoes and invasive snail species which help transmit waterborne parasites. Governments have spent decades trying to eradicate it, mostly without success, but the best chance today may be to set up biogas digesters to generate electricity or to mix the leaves with animal dung for fertiliser. But it is expensive to harvest, heavy to transport and the machines cost communities too much.

Sudanese diplomat Nagat Mubarak El Tayeb, who, when working for the Sudanese government, had been responsible for trying to control the hyacinth and other weeds, admitted it was almost impossible. 'At one time, it infested over 3,500 square kilometres of water. It blocked the light, it prevented fishing, it changed the flora and fauna, it made travelling on the river more expensive, and it reduced people's incomes and made them hungry and ill.'[6]

* * *

That link between human and plant health is seldom made but vital to understand, says Bukar Tijani, the UN's former Assistant Director-General for Agriculture. Not only are plant diseases causing vast yield losses, often leading to starvation and social unrest, but they are undermining the health of whole ecosystems and the people and animals who depend on them.[7]

The scale of crop losses due to pests is now phenomenal – and growing. There are gaps in the data, but entomologists and the UN's Food and Agriculture Organization have calculated that as much as half of all that is grown commercially may be eaten by pests, at a cost of more than $200 billion a year. 'Anything that reduces yields, especially in vulnerable places, can affect health. Each day, we witness a shocking number of threats to the well-being of our plants and, by extension, to our health, environment and economy,' says Tijani.

Tell that to Moqbal Hossain. I met him in his village in southern Bangladesh near Cox's Bazar, practically in tears at the damage done four nights previously to his small field of tomatoes by a one-centimetre-long caterpillar he had identified as *Tuta absoluta* or the tomato leafminer. It had fed voraciously through half the crop, burrowing into stalks and chomping on buds and fruit. He had reached for a herbicide but without success. 'This one is new. We had been warned of this but what could we do? These pests are getting stronger, I am sure,' he told me. 'We cannot stop them.'[8]

Tuta absoluta is one of the most economically devastating pests the world knows. Confined more or less harmlessly to the central highlands of Peru for millennia, it was not known to Western science until 1917, when English entomologist Edward Meyrick found one of the moths on a plant at an altitude of nearly 3,000 metres in Huancayo province. No one paid much attention when it began to spread across Latin America in the 1980s, but in 2006 everything changed when it reached Spain, probably transported in packing cases or farm equipment.

Since then it has spread nearly 800 kilometres a year south and east, first across Europe and then throughout Africa. It is now established in the Middle East, India, Bangladesh and Nepal, and inevitably it is on its way to China.

Some pests kill plants; others kill people indirectly. One of the more serious invasive pests circulating today is the fall armyworm (*Spodoptera frugiperda*), another moth that arrived from tropical America and then swept across Africa in 2017, from where it marched into Asia. It's estimated that this pest has the potential to cause maize yield losses approaching 30 per cent across twelve of Africa's maize-producing countries. After being reported in India in 2018, it was subsequently found in other countries in Asia, including Bangladesh, China, Indonesia, Laos, Myanmar, Nepal, the Philippines, Sri Lanka, Taiwan, Thailand and Vietnam.

These global plant pandemics, which take place mostly below the radar of the public, weaken human resistance to disease and make whole ecosystems vulnerable.[9] One of the few times a government took notice of an invasive species was in 1853. No one was greatly concerned when a few old vines turned yellow, withered and died in the French village of Pujaut near Avignon in the southern Rhône valley. But the following year the same thing happened. When examined, the vines were found to be rotting from top to bottom, but there was no evidence of what had harmed them.

By then it was too late to stop what became known as the great French vine plague. Over the next ten years the mysterious disease spread around France and crossed to Spain, Italy and beyond.

Nowhere was immune. Within twenty-five years around 600,000 hectares of vines had to be uprooted and burned.

The great biologist Louis Pasteur was called in and recommended using soil fungi to control the disease, but he was too far ahead of his time and was ignored; other scientists proposed flooding the vineyards in the winter months, even suggesting people bury live toads below the plants to soak up the mysterious poison.

Nothing worked. The French wine industry, the most important in the world at the time, was economically laid waste, and tens of thousands of impoverished farm labourers were forced to leave the countryside, many taking their skills and families to the Americas, where they established new wine industries.[10] It took a French government inquiry in 1869 to show how a millimetre-long aphid, known today as *Phylloxera vastatrix*, was responsible. How it reached Pujaut is unknown, but it probably hitchhiked from North America via London on cuttings which French vintners were using. There should have been no problem – American vines had long been grown in France – but it was thought that pathogens like phylloxera could not survive the long Atlantic sea voyage. It was the advent of fast steamships from the 1850s onwards which had allowed phylloxera to stay alive for longer, and then invade France and devastate the European wine industry.

The solution was eventually found by grafting French cuttings onto phylloxera-resistant American rootstock – an arrangement still fiercely debated today by wine purists. Just as most human diseases never really go away, phylloxera is now widespread around the world, with only parts of Chile and Australia free of the pest.[11]

* * *

Some invasions have been well intentioned but ecologically disastrous. Japanese knotweed, introduced in the nineteenth century to beautify European and North American gardens, is now rampant, crowding out native plants and causing billions of dollars' worth of damage a year, and is practically impossible to eradicate. Since its arrival in France in boxes of pottery from China in 2004, the Asian hornet has rapidly colonised most European countries, where it affects the pollination of crops and could be responsible for the loss of up to two-thirds of all honeybee colonies in infested areas.[12] Most tragic of all, perhaps, Burmese pythons invaded the Florida Everglades when a snake-breeding farm was hit by Hurricane Andrew in 1992. In thirty years they have overwhelmed the native wildlife, reducing populations of foxes, rabbits, raccoons and birds by up to 60 per cent.

Sometimes the damage was anticipated but judged acceptable in the wider interest. The Nile perch introduced by the British to Lake Victoria in 1954 to create a Ugandan fishing industry quickly made extinct around 200 species of gaudy little cichlids. Today the Nile perch is itself close to extinction in the lake, having been all but fished out. Many animals were introduced to eradicate other introduced ones, with doubly disastrous results for biodiversity. The voracious rosy wolfsnail was dispatched to many Pacific islands from Florida and Central America in the 1940s to try to reduce populations of the giant African snail – a creature which itself had been introduced earlier by French administrators to provide tasty bites for gourmands. Alas! The rosy snail eschewed the African snail, far preferring to dine on the many small local snails. After more than fifty species had been made extinct on the islands, a massive international effort by zoos has bred tens of thousands of tiny partula snails to introduce back to their homelands.

Sometimes the invading force is so great that nothing can be done. When Herman Merkel, chief forester of what is now the Bronx Zoo in New York, first saw American chestnut trees struggling with a fungal pathogen in 1904, he had no idea it would go on to kill 3–4 billion trees in just a few decades. The disease had arrived with infected Japanese chestnuts and devastated vast areas of the Eastern states in one of the greatest plant pandemics of modern times.

Farmers and conservationists mostly dislike these invaders and the changes they bring. Assumed to be bad, they are held responsible for declines and extinctions, costing trillions of dollars a year to control. Like marauding Vikings or Goths, they are attributed warlike, mostly masculine qualities, like aggression, domination and hostility, damned for growing too big or too fast, and accused of pushing out beloved animals like red squirrels and native bluebells.

Much of this is unfair, because the damage done by invasive species is mostly human-inflicted. Pests and pathogens depend on us to travel, and find niches when the climatic or other environmental conditions are right. As a general rule, they home in on where humans have settled, and take hold in disturbed places like the edge of fragmented forests, overfished rivers and places disturbed by pollution, fire, drought, flood, hurricanes and intensive farming.

Indeed, humans are reaping both the benefits and the disadvantages of invasions encouraged a hundred years ago. Daniel Simberloff, director of the Institute for Biological Invasions at the University of Tennessee, tells how in 1898 the US Department of Agriculture set up an Office of Plant and Seed Introductions, which paid American explorers to travel the world to seek out and bring back to the US 'economically useful' plants. Together these travellers introduced many of the plants that have made the US the world's prime food producer, including soya beans, pistachios, mangoes, dates and bamboo.

What they also brought back, however, were the parasites, pathogens, pests and weeds that came with the beneficial plants and animals, and which farmers and gardeners have been trying to eliminate ever since. By 1940, says Simberloff, there were about 800 introduced insect species alone in the US; by 1980 there were 1,350 and today there are well over 2,000. Europe now has around 14,000 established non-native species.

But gauging numbers and attributing costs is fraught. One major University College London study suggests that invasive species are responsible for the demise of 261 of the 782 animal species known to have become extinct since AD 1500 as well as 39 of the 153 plant species that have disappeared.[13] This is way ahead of natural extinctions, or ones caused by over-hunting or farming.

The escalating economic cost of invasive species and the plant diseases they bring is now forcing countries to pay attention. In Canada, where invasive insects like the emerald ash borer have ravaged hundreds of thousands of hectares of Ontario's forests and giant hogweed has taken over whole valleys in British Columbia, it costs farmers and foresters around $7.5 billion a year to manage.[14] Australia spends $4 billion a year controlling alien plants alone. In the US, where there are possibly 50,000 invasive species, it costs around $120 billion a year.[15] Back in 2008, economists calculated that invasive species cost six major countries including South Africa, Brazil and New Zealand more than $300 billion a year to manage – almost as much as they spent on military security. On their own, these interlopers may not make much difference, but taken together and over time they may reduce biodiversity to a point where economies suffer and extinctions take place.

Invasive species may have another, so far barely understood effect on biodiversity and, indirectly, human and plant health. The evidence is that most species are declining as a result of human activities and are being replaced by a much smaller number of the pushy new ones that thrive in human-altered environments. The end result, some botanists say, will be fewer species, less variety and complexity and more disease. Others, like the science writer Fred Pearce, argue that every part of nature is in the continual process of being changed by the arrival of new plants and diseases, and the newcomers actually strengthen it. Far from being a threat, they are invigorating nature. Rather than repel these modern invaders, we should welcome them and celebrate nature's changes.[16]

Leading German invasion ecologist Hanno Seebens sees alien species as increasingly important in the global evolutionary process. 'It is as if nature has been put on fast forward. The number of alien species … has increased continuously over the last two hundred years. with more than a third of all first introductions recorded between 1970 and 2014. There are no signs of a slowdown in their arrival, and we have to expect more new invasions in the near future.'[17]

But to understand just why these great changes in human and plant health were happening now, I needed to explore the underlying causes of change and find out what was driving them. This investigation was to take me from chicken farms in Africa to the slums of Bangladesh, by way of bushmeat markets in Congo. It started close to the North Pole.

PART II

THE DRIVERS OF DISEASE

We will now discuss in a little more detail the
struggle for existence.

Charles Darwin, *On the Origin of Species*, 1859

8

A FAREWELL TO ICE

It was 2012 and we were at 83.20N, 6.20E, just a few hundred kilometres from the North Pole. The air temperature was −3°C and the sea was close to freezing, but where was the ice? After steaming north from Svalbard inside the Arctic Circle for ten days, the *Arctic Sunrise* had met only small, thin, one- and two-year-old floes which melt and reform every year. No permanent ice? It was unheard of at this latitude.

Ice pilot Arne Sorensen, a weather-hardened, thoughtful Dane who had spent half his life sailing at both poles, barely believed what he was not seeing. Standing twenty metres up in the open crow's nest, with the ship pitching and rolling twenty-five degrees to port and starboard in the great Arctic Ocean swells, he was searching through the mist for ice thick enough for scientists to land on to do their experiments.

'Ice is like people. When young it's sharp and angular. The older it gets the rounder it is.'[1] He could have added that the deeper into polar ice you go, the more silent it becomes.

Visibility was just 200 metres but, using the ship's remote steering system, Sorensen inched the ice breaker forward. He managed only about fifteen kilometres that day but there was still no old ice. Indeed, the further north we went, the more the young floes were piled up and compressed in fantastic shapes and shades of grey and blue, cracking, rumbling and groaning as we nudged them aside or climbed over them. Two polar bears on our port side lifted their heads but resumed hunting.

How different this voyage was from ones Sorensen had made when young, he said. By mid-September, the leading edge of the Arctic ice cap would normally be hundreds of kilometres further south. About 600,000 square kilometres more ice had already melted. 'Now we are close to the pole. This is the frontline of climate change. I am certain it is because we burn fossil fuels. It is sad to observe that we are capable of changing the planet to such a degree. You wonder where it will end.'[2]

Down in the galley, Cambridge University sea ice researcher Nick Toberg, who had analysed underwater ice thickness data collected by British nuclear submarine HMS *Tireless* in 2004 and 2007, was equally astonished. He explained the importance of the sea ice:

It is a lid on the planet that regulates the temperature. By taking it off you are warming it. Temperatures [everywhere] depend on it. What we are seeing is staggering. It's disturbing, scary, that we have physically changed the face of the planet so much. We have about 4 million square kilometres of sea ice. If that goes in the summer months that's about the same as adding twenty years of CO_2 at current [human-caused] rates into the atmosphere. That's how vital the Arctic sea ice is. In the 1970s we had 8 million square kilometres of sea ice. That has been halved. We need it in the summer. It has never decreased like this before. We knew the ice was getting thinner but no one expected we'd lose this much so soon. We broke the record by a lot.[3]

* * *

When temperatures rise, everything changes and disease arrives. As the thick ice melts and the seas and the air warm, so new life arrives in Arctic waters. Minke, bottlenose, fin and sperm whales are heading north, even as grizzly bears, white-tailed deer, coyotes and other animals and birds expand their range into boreal forests to the south.

But the geography of disease is also changing as novel pathogens affecting plants, animals and humans increase their range. New beetles are heading north and devastating Siberian forests, Alaskan mammals are struggling as new ticks arrive and human habitations in northern Norway are infested by new insects.

In Alaska, where winter warming has increased by nearly 4°C in sixty years, the whole ecosystem is undergoing change. The sea ice is breaking up earlier than it used to, causing changes in the amount of phytoplankton – the minute organisms that drift around in water currents – at the bottom of the food chain. This has knock-on effects on fish and bird populations. Lakes are changing size, marine heat waves are becoming more frequent and more intense, and mammals must seek new food sources. The author Edward Struzik reports 'a plethora of deadly and debilitating diseases' striking reindeer in Scandinavia and Russia, musk oxen on Banks and Victoria islands in Arctic Canada and polar bears and seals off the coast of Alaska.[4]

New pathogens are turning up everywhere. They may be strange pests in Malawian maize fields, a novel fungal infection appearing in the ear of a Japanese woman, an unidentified insect killing trees in Russia, or a new bacterium shrivelling the fruit of lemon trees in Florida.[5]

I called Daniel Brooks, a bacteriologist at the Harold W. Manter Laboratory of Parasitology at the University of Nebraska State Museum. He and his colleagues' studies show that with global heating, pathogens are jumping more frequently from one host to another. He argues that climate will soon be fuelling pandemics and we can expect a succession of unpredictable human, animal and plant disease outbreaks. 'We rarely have an idea where the next [pathogen] will pop up. All we know is that they are better at finding us than we have been [at] finding them.'[6]

Brooks places climate change and disease in historical and ecological context. 'When the climate is stable,' he says, 'species tend to be isolated and specialised. But when it is volatile, as it is now becoming, environments change and this creates opportunities for new species to colonise and evolve. Throughout the past 15,000 years, advances in civilisation – agriculture, domestication, the flourishing of cities and globalisation – have all been accompanied by increasing disease risk. But never before has the human population been larger, living at such high densities and so hyperconnected. We are now approaching a storm of spiralling disease risks.'[7]

Past pandemics, he says, largely arose at times of climate shifts that destabilised human populations and forced migration, famines and conflict. They then subsided with the return of climate stability. So long as climate change continues to stir up the biosphere, pathogens will continue to move between humans, farmed animals and wildlife. 'The planet is a minefield of evolutionary accidents waiting to happen. Now we are in a period of accelerating climate activity, we should expect more emerging diseases. It is these emerging diseases, made more likely by climate change, which then exacerbate poverty, famine, drought, conflict and migration.'[8]

Climate change, he emphasised, does not produce disease itself; rather, it is a 'multiplier', increasing and speeding up the threat of diseases emerging. When temperatures rise or fall, when the rains are heavier or a drought lasts longer, then the conditions for life change and the insects, bats or ticks that often carry the pathogens of diseases like malaria, Rift Valley fever, cholera and dengue are likely to move geographically.

Far from being linked definitively to a single host, as was thought for many years, Brooks and colleagues are showing that viruses and bacteria can and do switch hosts frequently, with the result that new diseases will inevitably emerge or old ones flare up more easily with climate change. They suggest that we have a crisis of emerging infectious disease, with known pathogens becoming more dangerous than before, appearing somewhere new or infecting new hosts, changing both the movement of pathogens and the impact they have on humans and animals.

Other work suggests that climate and land use changes over the coming decades will together produce many new opportunities for viruses to jump between species and cross to humans. At the moment, says Colin Carlson at the Center for Global Health

Science and Security at Georgetown University, some 10,000 virus species have the capacity to infect us, but the vast majority circulate silently and unrecognised in wild mammals. His models simulate how 3,139 species will share viruses and create new spillover risk hotspots. In the warmer, physically degraded world that we are creating, species will naturally converge in new combinations at high altitude, in places of high biodiversity and where human populations are concentrated, most likely in Asia and Africa. Mammals like bats will encounter other mammals for the first time, potentially sharing thousands of viruses. This ecological transition may already be underway, he says.[9]

The implications of research like that of Brooks and Carlson are enormous, says Canadian-French ecologist Timothée Poisot. 'It shows that there isn't a "climate" future and a "pandemics" future, there's just a future made of synergistic effects.'[10]

When it comes to warming, the ecological process goes roughly like this: the temperature rises, which affects rainfall and humidity, wind patterns and the amount of sunshine; this increases the severity of cyclones, floods, droughts and heatwaves, which in turn affect the survival, dispersal and reproduction of pathogens that are linked to outbreaks of cholera, typhoid, filariasis, leptospirosis, malaria, yellow fever and a host of other diseases.[11]

Changes in a warming world are throwing up many medical surprises. Two years after I joined Arne Sorensen in the crow's nest of the *Arctic Sunrise*, the far past returned to northern Russia with an anthrax outbreak that killed a twelve-year-old boy and infected dozens of semi-nomadic reindeer herders and their animals. A heatwave with temperatures reaching an unprecedented 37°C had part-melted the permafrost and exposed a reindeer corpse that had died of the disease many years before and been buried barely a metre deep in the frozen ground. More than forty people were taken to hospital.

Until then it had barely occurred to me that a warming climate might disinter dormant but still active pathogens. Viruses and bacteria can 'live' for millennia when frozen, and no one has much idea what else may be entombed in icy soils and glaciers to be released with heating. We have not had long to wait for more evidence. In the past five years, the European Space Agency has found hundreds of ancient microorganisms resistant to antibiotics in the Alaskan permafrost, and Chinese hunters have isolated thirty-three ancient and previously unknown viruses dating back at least 11,000 years inside Tibetan glaciers and ice samples in Greenland and elsewhere. There will surely be many more similar discoveries.

* * *

The unexpected arrived at the luxurious home of retired Michigan insurance worker Florence Smith in the Upper Keys area of Key Largo in Monroe County, Florida, on 2 August 2020. That morning she woke with a fever, which soon turned to vomiting and a rash. A friend took her to a hospital brimming with first-wave Covid-19 patients, where she was eventually diagnosed with dengue, a nasty viral infection she had heard about but paid scant attention to because it is widely thought of as a disease of Africa.

Florence should have known better. On its web page, Monroe County claims to be 'ground zero for experiencing the impacts of global climate change and sea level rise'.[12] The county comprises the chain of flat, low-lying islands of the Florida Keys and is one of the most vulnerable places in the world both to sea-level rise and hurricanes. Many of its streets are regularly flooded, and people frequently say they are considering leaving or raising their homes. After all, the Key West sea level has officially risen ten centimetres since 2000, and by 2040 the sea is expected to rise a further fifteen to thirty centimetres, which would be catastrophic for nearly everyone who lives there.[13]

I spoke to Dr Mark Whiteside, Monroe's director of medicine, in the middle of the Covid-19 crisis. 'Climate change is affecting us hard, both physically and medically,' he said. 'We are grappling with rising seas and not one, but two completely new health epidemics. We expect hurricanes and sea level rise, but no one thought of Covid-19 or dengue.'[14]

Whiteside lives in Key West, the southernmost city in the continental United States, and has been studying infectious diseases there for nearly thirty years. He summarised the evolution of dengue in Florida. Until 2009 it was more or less unknown in the Keys. There had been a small, limited outbreak of a mild form in South Florida but everyone recovered and the disease, which he thought had been brought in by travellers, then disappeared. But in April 2020 it returned with a vengeance and, critically, was found to be transmitting locally. The mosquitoes were now breeding in the Keys and infecting an area much further north in the Upper Keys.

'I fully expect dengue to return year after year now. It will increase for certain. It won't go away. There's always a possibility that it becomes more severe.' I asked him if he thought climate change had brought it to the Keys. 'Global warming is out of control in my opinion, but I say the reason dengue is so successful is that it has adapted itself to humans. Warming may be just one factor.'[15]

Dengue is carried by two species of mosquitoes, *Aedes aegypti* and *Aedes albopictus*. It kills about 25,000 people a year but infects around 500 million in 100 countries, of which around 500,000 cases develop into severe illness. It is perfectly suited to spread fast in a warming, more humid, urbanised world. Cases are doubling every decade or so, and by 2050 it is expected to have spread from its heartlands in South Asia to become endemic in Southern Mediterranean countries like Spain, Portugal, Italy and Greece, as well as much of Japan, China and Australia. Just a slight rise in temperature and rainfall could see outbreaks in cities like Paris, New York and London.

But despite many warnings from epidemiologists, dengue invariably catches governments unprepared. Small-scale epidemics triggered by returning travellers have broken out across Europe for a decade, but so fast is it spreading that it's probably only a matter of time before the mosquitoes start breeding and the disease establishes itself in Italy or Spain. When it arrived in Thailand in 2019, 100,000 people were infected and hundreds died. Honduras and Costa Rica both declared an emergency the same year, when thousands were infected. In 2021 it ravaged cities in China, India, Pakistan and Nepal.[16]

Global heating is far from dengue's only driver – population growth and the worldwide move to cities are also important – but it is clearly linked to planetary heating, say the Oxford University geographers who in 2019 crunched temperature, population, medical and economic data and forecast that half the world could be living in places where *Aedes aegypti* breeds by 2050.[17]

Mosquitoes carry dengue, malaria and chikungunya, but blood-sucking ticks, black flies, sand flies, midges and fleas are equally sensitive to temperature and rainfall changes and are able to transmit human pathogens more easily in the warmer, wetter weather most of the world is experiencing with global warming. Other diseases that are transmitted in water, like cholera, salmonellosis and giardia, are also more likely to break out in warming temperatures.[18]

* * *

I had not appreciated before how sensitive all life is to rainfall and temperature, and therefore how even a small shift in the climate can change the ecological balance and trigger disease.

When Norwegian researchers studied thousands of plague outbreaks in the Middle Ages and compared them to climate data from tree-ring records, they found that the recurring waves of the Black Death pandemic invariably followed a warm summer in central Asia that came after a wet spring. They also pinned the blame not on black rats, which do not thrive in those conditions, but on gerbils whose fleas carry the plague bacteria and which must have hitched a ride to Europe with travellers along the Silk Road.

Others have shown how a warming climate favours insects, pests, ticks and fleas which often carry plant and animal pathogens. The IPCC, the UN body that assesses the evidence of climate change, reports how half the world's insects can be expected to 'substantially' increase their ranges over the next few decades, leading to crop losses, animal diseases and probably global food shortages.

The number of malaria cases in any one year in Kenya and Ethiopia is directly linked to rainfall and high temperatures in critical months. Severe outbreaks of Murray Valley encephalitis, caused by a mosquito-borne virus, invariably occur after heavy rainfall and flooding in South Australia. Big rains in Canada always seem to lead to E. coli and campylobacter outbreaks and waterborne diseases in Bangladesh consistently peak in the monsoon months. From bluetongue disease in sheep to Rift Valley fever in camels, researchers say that climate is now determining the spread of disease.

The obvious reason is that warming temperatures give many insects a competitive advantage. It speeds up their rates of reproduction and development and improves their chances of survival as well as increasing their range. We humans may think that a 1°C rise in temperature is not much, but for a pathogen in an insect it may be substantial because they're so much more sensitive to climate.

Our own sensitivity to temperature is also remarkably limited. We disguise it with technology, light fires and put on the air conditioning, but we are nearly as vulnerable as any insect. The human body has evolved to work within a very narrow range of body temperature – in our case 36°C to 37.5°C – and anything outside that can be dangerous.

* * *

I chose to go to Manila, the megacity capital of the Philippines, to see how a warming climate was affecting health in an urban area of 13 million or more densely packed people. This is the most exposed country in the world to typhoons and tropical storms. In November 2013 Typhoon Haiyan, known locally as Yolanda, had brewed up 500 kilometres to the east near the equator. It rapidly developed into a superstorm and slammed into the city of Tacloban, where it flattened almost every building, killed 6,300, triggered diseases and traumatised millions of people. It was the greatest storm ever to have made landfall anywhere in the world, with winds gusting at over 300 kilometres per hour.

Physicists today can quite quickly identify the links between human-induced climate change and heatwaves, drought, flood and other specific catastrophes, but the Haiyan disaster was in 2013 and scientists were cautious to do so. Nevertheless, it made instinctive sense. Storms receive their energy from the ocean, so it is logical that they would get stronger, and perhaps also more frequent, with warmer seas.

I headed straight to PAGASA, the government body which tracks storms and warns Filipinos of oncoming weather-related danger. It was a steaming 34°C outside and raining heavily. I was met by Jean, a cheerful young meteorologist. I asked her whether she thought Haiyan had been a natural or a human-made disaster. She laid out the bare facts: 'Climate change is heating up the Pacific Ocean where the typhoons start, making them move faster and more powerfully. Climate change does not produce its own impacts,' she insisted. 'Rather, it amplifies, or magnifies what is already there.' She called it a 'threat multiplier'.

We see here in Manila that there has been a significant increase [in the last thirty years] in the number of hot days and warm nights and a decreasing trend in the number of cold days and cold nights. Both maximum and minimum temperatures are getting warmer. Extreme rainfall events are becoming more common and the number of heatwaves is more frequent. In most parts the intensity of rainfall is increasing. The number of cyclones is less than it was, but they are getting stronger and more dangerous. The number of people now affected by disease and flooding is growing.[19]

The government's raw statistics certainly suggested that the region's typhoons were getting stronger. From 1947 to 1960, the most powerful one to hit the country was Amy in December 1951, whose highest wind speed was recorded in Cebu at 240 kilometres per hour. From 1961 to 1980, the highest wind speed recorded was 275 kilometres per hour, in October 1970. Since then the highest wind speed has soared to 320 kilometres per hour, recorded during Typhoon Durian (Reming) in November to December 2006.

Three kilometres away in Barangay (district) Kamuning, I met Joshua and Maria Alvarez and their young family. The previous year, their two-bedroom ground-floor apartment had been flooded when a storm dumped thirty-eight centimetres of rain in a few hours and the local reservoir had overflowed. Several large areas of the capital were flooded with muddy waters up to three metres deep and, with hundreds of others, they had fled to a flyover. Now they were starting life again in a better-protected flat. In the wake of the disaster, Belinda, one of their children, had caught a respiratory disease; another, Keanu, had diarrhoea. Both illnesses were a result of the floods, said Maria.

In one of Manila's new suburbs, I also met Denis Posadas, a young technologist and climate specialist who had moved his young family out of the city centre for health reasons. 'It is getting unbearable. Tens of thousands of people in Manila live in shanty towns that are in the way of the floods. These people will be the most vulnerable. Climate change is also making some places here uninhabitable, hotter than the human body can stand. It will slow down economic growth, trigger new poverty traps and create hotspots of hunger,' he said. Posadas was resigned to ill health: 'These days 32°C is common and lots of people still do not have fridges – so food goes off and people get ill. Heat brings mosquitoes and fevers. I've noticed how when temperatures are really high, evaporation is greater in the reservoirs, which means there is less water, and mosquitoes.'[20]

When Haiyan hit in 2013, I was in Doha, covering the COP 19 climate talks. Also in attendance was Yeb Sano, the Filipino government's young climate-change diplomat. He had been trying to get news of his brother and his family, who lived in the stricken Tacloban. Memorably, he had addressed the global meeting and broken down in tears.

Now he was resolute and more certain than ever that his country was in danger:

The scientists tell us it will probably get 4°C warmer. That means everything will be compromised, from health and food and energy to settlements. We are just not ready. The challenge is too huge. I cannot imagine what would happen if a typhoon the strength of Yolanda hit Manila or the second city, Cebu. It would be a global disaster. It will take us twenty years to recover from Yolanda as it is. We lost one million homes then. Rich countries tell us to become climate resilient. We agree, but who pays? We have received possibly $5 million from the World Bank for studies [on how] to adapt to climate change, and that is all.[21]

To double-check how disease follows Manila's regular heatwaves and annual flooding, I dropped into a Quezon City health clinic. Dr Angel Fernandez was at the sharp end of the city's health and she counted off on her fingers the most obvious health impacts. 'Dengue. Allergies. Leptospirosis. Heart disease. Skin and fungal infections. Heat stress. Depression. Tetanus. Water diseases.' Would she say these were climate diseases, I asked? 'Of course. But especially the heat.'

* * *

Heatwaves are not just lasting longer and becoming more intense in the tropics but are also more frequent and affect many more vulnerable people in northern latitudes and in rich countries. By one count, global heatwave exposure grew from 40 billion person-days in 1983 to 119 billion person-days in 2016. By another, the number of heatwaves that last for four days or more is growing, as are the number of days when the temperature reaches 50°C. In a third study, it was found that more than one in four of the US population suffered from the effects of extreme heat and that 1 billion people, or one in seven in the world, could expect to do so if temperatures rise a further 1°C.[22] A record 175 million people endured heatwaves in 2015 alone. One study of more than 13,000 cities worldwide found that people are now exposed to three times as many extreme heat days as they were in the 1980s, due partly to the growing urban population and partly to rising temperatures.[23]

But global heating is far from uniform, and some cities are more affected than others. Dhaka, the capital of Bangladesh, has had some of the highest rises in extreme heat days. Others, like Manila, Shanghai, Hanoi, Bangkok and Yangon, have all experienced increases.[24] Aside from latitude and distance to the sea or to mountains, the level of heating depends too on the size of the city, whether it has many cooler parks and gardens, the materials it has been built with and the number of cars it has.

* * *

I met Devinder in 2014 in the city of Bodh Gaya during one of India's recurrent heatwaves. All northern India was scorching but Bihar, one of the poorest states, was said to be experiencing its hottest-ever spring. The local Met office had recorded a temperature of 44°C the previous week and this was the third deadly heatwave in just over two months.

Devinder was one of a group of day labourers. Stripped to the waist, they had started work wheelbarrowing sand and gravel for the foundations of a house at 5 a.m. They had been told they did not need to work after 10 a.m., but now it was midday and they had carried on because they needed the money.

He looked sixty, said he was just twenty-eight, and lived in a village one hour out of the city. He was exhausted. Two of his friends had gone to hospital when dizzy with what was probably heat stress. One man from his village had died yesterday. 'My small wheat crop has failed. My wife is pregnant and we need food. I have no option now but to work in the city because it is cooler here. Farming work is too hot.'

India is notorious for its heat, which regularly kills thousands of the poorest people. But the spring of 2022 was exceptionally hot across tens of thousands of square kilometres, with a series of heatwaves between March and July. As temperatures hit 50°C in places and cities issued hundreds of red alerts for people to stay at home, crops were ruined, dairy herds stopped producing milk, public fountains ran dry and factories ground to a halt when electricity grids failed.

I spoke by phone with a doctor at the city hospital, which was turning people away, saying its air conditioning had failed and it could not handle all the heat victims. 'A temperature of 43°C is impossible to live with for more than a few days. Now it is 46ºC. How can we endure this? This is like the end of the world. We got through the Covid pandemic but now we are dying of heat; every year it gets worse.'

Heat stress is now a global problem. Most of the northern hemisphere experienced simultaneous heatwaves throughout 2022. Pulses of hot air coming off the Sahara, Arabian and Gobi deserts started earlier than usual in March and continued well into the northern hemisphere's summer, engulfing cities and breaking temperature records across North America, Europe and China.

The long-term health consequences of life in a world experiencing prolonged and ever more intense heatwaves is barely known. But heat is known to kill and affect vulnerable people in many ways. Aside from heat stress, heart collapse and kidney failure, it is associated with crime, depression and suicide, and has been blamed for war and rising political tensions.[25]

One analysis of more than 2,300 European weather disaster records from 1981 to 2010 suggested that the number of people dying each year from excessive heat would rise from 2,700 now to 151,000 in fifty years. A similar World Health Organization study predicted that by 2050 heatwaves could kill around 255,000 people around the world each year.[26]

Besides, it's not heat alone that is dangerous. Anyone who has spent time in the tropics will tell you that heat combined with humidity is the hardest to live with. At a certain point there is so much moisture in the air that even if you are sweating profusely, your body cannot cool down. Humid heat is possibly the most underestimated direct, local risk of climate change, says Radley Horton, the Columbia University professor who led a US National Oceanic and Atmosphere (NOAA) study which showed that extreme heat across the world had tripled in recent decades.[27]

Heat can be measured in different ways. A thermometer reading gives only the heat of the air, but a reading from one placed in the shade and covered in a wet cloth combines heat and humidity. This is known as a 'wet bulb' reading and is usually far lower. An air temperature of over 40°C (104°F) may be bearable in super-dry desert heat, but a much lower temperature would be highly dangerous if it were both hot and humid. Any 'wet bulb' temperature over 32°C is defined as an 'extreme risk' for people with health conditions like respiratory or heart diseases and for the elderly, as well as those working outdoors. At 30°C in humid places like Lagos or Manila, even the healthiest people, relaxing in the shade and with an endless supply of water, cannot stop themselves from overheating. What starts with a headache and sweating moves quickly on to dizziness, fainting, vomiting, confusion and anxiety and ends up as a coma, affecting nearly every organ and increasing the risk of strokes, seizures and heart attacks. A wet bulb temperature of 35°C is the upper physiological limit of humans, the point when the body can no longer cool itself by sweating. Even the fittest people can die in a few hours.[28]

Tom Matthews and colleagues at Loughborough University in the UK analysed weather data from around the world and found that the frequency of wet bulb temperatures between 27°C and 35°C had doubled since 1979. People in the Gulf, India, Pakistan, the US and Mexico are most at risk. In 2020 the deadly wet bulb temperature of 35°C was recorded for the first time at Jacobabad in Pakistan and at Ras Al Khaimah, northeast of Dubai in the United Arab Emirates (UAE).

While some people facing extreme heat and humidity can adapt by switching on the AC, plants have no chance and the result of rising temperatures is not just failed crops but malnutrition and diseases of poverty.[29] Staples like maize, wheat and soybeans are more sensitive to temperature and rainfall than most animals and, say researchers from NASA, harvests could be drastically hit far sooner than anyone thought only thirty years ago. For every 1°C rise in average global temperature, wheat and rice yields are expected to decline by 6 and 10 per cent respectively.

Climate scientist Chandni Singh in Delhi poses the moral question that heatwaves raise and which governments ignore. In April 2022 a fierce, unseasonal heatwave had spread across most of India and Pakistan, affecting 1 billion mostly poor people with temperatures of 44°C or higher. Singh had to be out in the scorching heat for three hours. 'I waited for an air-conditioned bus but it was full, so I took another, which was not air-conditioned. After an hour-long ride, I was home. Despite plenty of water and a cool home to come to, I'm still feeling the after-effects of heat exposure a day later. Fatigue and desiccation, physical and mental,' she said.

> But where do we go from here? Across the subcontinent we have a history of living with heat. We keep water cool in earthen pots, vendors splash water on pavements, water is kept for anyone to drink from in public spaces. But these are coping measures at best, effective for short periods of heat exposure only. Coping lulls us into believing we can deal with this. But as days and nights get hotter, coping can only get us so far.
>
> But sitting in an air-conditioned room as it boils outside, it is almost unthinkable to consider mitigation, to consider switching off the AC. Those who can cool will cool; those who can't can only cope. I feel angry that the best we are doing is leaving the most vulnerable people behind.[30]

* * *

I first visited Malawi in March 2002 during a terrible drought which had left 80 per cent of the small Southern African country of 12 million people hungry and many thousands dead. Malawi was then – and still is – is one of the poorest countries in the world. Few people there earn more than $1 per day and nearly everyone depends on a single rainy season to grow a staple crop of maize. As such it is acutely vulnerable to rising temperatures and rainfall.

I travelled between health clinics, hospitals and feeding centres, trying to understand how a famine could happen at the same time as hundreds of millions of people in Britain and other countries were overweight. It was distressing. Wherever I went, there was shocking destitution, malnutrition and death. In one hospital at Nambuma, a small town about fifty kilometres northwest of the capital, Lilongwe, many of the women and children said they were from a place called Gumbi.

'Why is it so bad there?' I asked a government health official called Patrick Kamzitu.

'Let's go and see,' he said.

You get to Gumbi from Nambuma by track, past a huge brick church built a hundred years ago by the White Fathers missionaries and a football pitch, and through what should be fields of two-metre-tall swaying maize. Gumbi consisted of about seventy mud-built, straw-thatched houses. The place was deserted and many structures had no roofs. A few women sat under a tree, their infants listless. A tired-looking man introduced himself as 'Mr Jamu, the chief'.

Gumbi had nothing, he told me. No shops, no food and no assets beyond a few bicycles and ox carts. There was a single book in the village of about three hundred people, but there was no electricity or TV, no generator, no health clinic or school, and everyone was hungry. Gumbi had been hit particularly hard by the drought, he said, because everyone was desperately poor and few people had skills other than growing maize or tobacco. The village was empty, because in times of hunger people left to seek work elsewhere in the tobacco plantations, but the drought had ruined that crop, too. Now they were looking for any work they could in the capital, Lilongwe.

Parents had taken children out of school to save money, and others were cutting the few remaining trees to make charcoal, collecting wild foods and leaves and berries, praying for rains that they knew would not come for months, or for food aid to arrive. Some just waited for the end. Many children showed signs of oedema, one of the signs of extreme malnutrition. Those who remained did what they always do in a major drought: they sold anything they could.

Today a three-year-long drought would most likely be auto-matically attributed to climate change, but it was not too hard to see that at its core, this was a man-made famine. The IMF and donor countries, including the UK, had told the Malawian government to sell off its grain reserves because they were expensive to maintain; the EU had mistakenly said that only a little food would be needed in the case of a local disaster and rich traders had bought and hoarded food and were now selling it at excessive prices.

I sat with the village elders and asked them whether the drought was unusual. Without prompting, they all said not just that it was an unusual drought but that nowadays the rains came at different times. Droughts were cyclical and came regularly, and they had coping mechanisms, but they could not remember anything so bad. There was no mention of climate change, which was barely on the UN or any political agenda.

Since 2002 I have been back to Gumbi and Malawi nearly every year. Patrick Kamzitu, the young health worker who showed me around in 2002 and who regularly visits twelve other villages and farms his own patch of land, has seen the changes in twenty years. 'Not only are droughts more frequent, but there are more hot days and nights and the rains are less predictable. It's getting harder to know when to plant and harvest the crops, harder to get out of poverty and almost impossible to achieve good health,' he told me.

Studies by the World Bank and others now back up what I heard over and over again in the villages of Malawi, Tanzania, Zambia, Mozambique and Kenya. They all report steadily rising temperatures, more floods and more intense rains and droughts. The growing seasons have become shorter, the yields smaller, and, despite a massive programme to eliminate it with bed nets and sprays, the prevalence of malaria is growing. Climate change may not be directly causing the droughts and floods that Gumbi and other villages are experiencing, but it is exacerbating natural phenomena, pushing much of the country to the brink of catastrophe.

The UN Food and Agriculture Organization has warned that for the first time in almost two decades the number of undernourished people has begun to rise, climbing to more than 400 million in Africa and Asia.[31] Worse will follow, they fear, if temperatures keep rising. They anticipate maize yields dropping 24 per cent – with drastic implications for hundreds of millions of people in Southern Africa who depend on a single crop – and slightly smaller drops for rice and soybeans, which feed nearly half the world's people and animals. The good news, they said, was that South Asia, the

Southern US, Mexico and parts of South America would be able to grow wheat for longer.

Climate change is not the only factor in Malawi's poverty and continuing malnutrition, but Felix Pensulo Phiri, Malawi's director of nutrition, told me that it acts as a multiplier, increasing the risk. 'Temperatures here are rising; there are more frequent floods and droughts. Drought not only leads to food shortages, which result in malnutrition, but also to more malaria. We anticipate more and more environmental health challenges relating to climate change because of the increasing population.'[32]

Back in the fields of Gumbi and Nambuma, farmers have one more problem to face. Three years ago the rains were particularly heavy and the following year their maize crop was devastated. Try as they might with insecticides, they could not stop this strange black worm chomping through their crops. It looked like the dreaded fallarmy worm, an invasive moth that has swept through Bangladesh, China, Indonesia, Laos, Myanmar, Nepal, the Philippines, Sri Lanka, Taiwan, Thailand and Vietnam in the past twenty years, but government entomologists who inspected it said it was something different.

These days the research is coming thick and fast. Changing temperatures and rainfall across Africa are now expected to increase yellow fever deaths by up to 25 per cent by 2050,[33] and force 100 million people into the extreme poverty by 2030, making them more vulnerable to health problems.[34] The *Lancet* did not mince its words when it said in 2019: 'Every child born today will have their health defined by climate change. By their 71st birthday, their physical and mental health will be likely burdened by other hazards, such as food shortages, the spread of diseases from insects, droughts, floods and wildfires.'[35]

Climate change is not a disease, but the extra heat, the sea level rises, the more intense storms and the new infections that it enables will over 100 years surely kill far more people than Covid-19, heart disease, air pollution, cholera, malaria and HIV/Aids combined if it is not addressed. The people most affected now are those in heat-stressed, poorer countries. But as patterns of disease change, crops fail, cities flood and drainage systems become overwhelmed, there will be no escape. Everyone will experience the health effects, whether heat, infections or storms.

Sometimes it needs a banker to deliver home truths. Mark Carney, the former Governor of the Bank of England, has grasped what is at stake: 'You cannot self-isolate from climate. That is not an option. We cannot retreat and wait out climate change. It will just get worse. When you look at it from a human mortality perspective, it will be the equivalent of a coronavirus crisis every year from the middle of this century, and every year, not just a one-off event. So it is an issue that needs to be addressed now.'[36]

9

TRADING PLACES

The Iziko South African Museum in Cape Town is a wonder of nature, a collection of over a million objects which together trace the whole span of evolution. Here are ancient cave art and the oldest-known human footprints, the bones of 200-million-year-old mammals and some of the world's oldest stone tools, as well as 700-million-year-old fossils and modern-day insects and fish.

Rarely seen, because it is tucked away in a drawer in one of the colonial-era buildings in Queen Victoria Street, is a specimen of a small frog whose relatives may have unwittingly changed the course of natural history. With its smooth, plump body and blotched, olive-grey skin, the African clawed frog, officially known as *Xenopus laevis*, is no beauty. But this tongueless, toothless, fast-breeding and secretive creature, with its cheeky face and wide mouth, is a star of human medicine.

Not only is the African clawed frog long-lived, making it popular with researchers who use it to study immunity and embryology, but it has evolved to survive just about anywhere. The French like to eat its legs, it has been sent into space by the Russians, and it has been experimented on by schoolchildren and Nobel Prize-winners alike.

Its greatest claim to fame is that for around forty years between the early 1930s and 1960s it was the world's most accurate and reliable human pregnancy tester. Who knows how it ever came to be suspected, but in 1929 British experimental biologist and writer

Lancelot Hogben was working with others on hormones at Cape Town University when they found that if a tiny bit of urine from a pregnant woman were injected into the hind leg of a female *X. laevis*, the frog would invariably spawn tiny eggs within twelve or so hours.[1]

In just a few years, the 'Hogben test', as it became known, was the gold-standard, 99.98 per cent accurate, fastest human pregnancy test available anywhere in the Western world. Tens of thousands of African clawed frogs were bred in farms by the South African government and entrepreneurs and shipped alive every year to laboratories, hospitals and pharmacies in the US, Canada and the UK. Once there, the technicians would inject a mature female frog with a urine sample and would soon get a result. Because the test didn't require the sacrifice of the animal, it was doubly popular with growing animal welfare movements.

But there was an unintended – in this case catastrophic – consequence of this live animal trade. Having done their work, many of the frogs were then given by institutions and pharmacies to the fast-growing pet trade, which in turn sold them on to households for a few cents each. Invariably, many also escaped from ponds and rivers and began interbreeding wherever there was water and suitable conditions. Today there are colonies of African clawed frogs everywhere from Maine to Madrid, and in nearly every aquarium.

This is where the problems began. The frog can carry on its skin the virulent chytrid fungus. This is harmless to the frog itself but microscopic bacterial spores can be shed in water and embed themselves in the skin of many amphibians, where they reproduce before returning to the water to infect new hosts. The disease, known as Batrachochytrium dendrobatidis or Bd, then chews through the flesh of other frogs, toads, newts and salamanders and gives them heart attacks.

In a little over thirty years the global trade in clawed frogs, first for medicine and research and later for the pet trade, devastated wild populations in the rainforests of Panama and Central America, and later in the US and Australia, Ecuador, Venezuela, New Zealand

and Spain. By the 1990s chytrid had spread to every continent except Antarctica. Populations of amphibians have since been found to be crashing in a global pandemic which makes Covid-19, Spanish flu and Ebola all look relatively mild.

Chytrid is one of the most serious diseases in the world, likely to have already destroyed more biodiversity than any other single disease.[2] Of the approximately 7,800 known amphibian species, more than 1,300 have been tested for chytrid and more than 700 have been found to be infected. Several hundred species are known to have been made extinct by it in the past thirty years, and thousands more are classed as 'threatened', with many of the rest in decline. Thanks to the global trade in clawed frogs, mass die-offs have been recorded in populations of salamanders, newts, toads and frogs. What is worse is that this ongoing amphibian pandemic shows no signs of stopping.

But only now have the secondary consequences of the trade been firmly connected to a change in human health. Researchers in Costa Rica have documented how when the frogs died off, there was a surge in the population of insects which the amphibians would have eaten, and a drop in the population of snakes which would have eaten the frogs. The net result may have been fewer snakebites but, more ominously, they identified a surge in human malaria cases.

* * *

The impact of the wildlife trade on the rest of nature is hard to judge accurately because it is both local and international, legal and illegal, and ranges from the organised criminal poaching of rhinos in Africa and tigers in Bangladesh to individual hunters trapping single pangolins or antelopes for the pot and the export of tens of thousands of songbirds for the international pet trade. Add in the unregulated mass breeding of snakes, crocodiles and other species for traditional medicine and fashion, and the newer practice of wildlife farms, which breed exotic animals for food and medical testing, and it is unsurprising that governments haven't a clue how much wildlife is traded, let alone how far it affects health.

To get some idea of its scale, I checked with the most authoritative sources I could find. There was no agreement on what even counted as wildlife and there was a wealth of overlapping figures and different ways to count. The US government's Centers for Disease Control and Prevention (CDC) estimated in 2006 that 40,000 live primates, 4 million live birds, 640,000 live reptiles and 350 million live tropical fish are traded globally each year.[3] Meanwhile, the Consortium for Conservation Medicine, one of the founding groups of the EcoHealth Alliance, has argued that more than 1 billion live animals are imported every year into the United States alone, with most going to the pet and food trade.[4]

Whichever way it is counted, the global trade in wild animals is vast and must be a significant factor in the worldwide decline of species. But is it also a global health risk, as many conservation and wildlife groups claim? It's important to know, because the best science suggests that one quarter of the mammals in the wildlife trade harbour 75 per cent of all known zoonotic viruses, meaning that the larger the trade, the more vulnerable people will be to new parasites, viruses and funguses to which they have not previously been exposed. In other words, the chances of wildlife directly or indirectly infecting humans grows with every contact between humans and wild animals.[5]

Complicating matters further is the fact that the trade in wild animals is a political football, with arguments flying between conservationists, industries, governments and indigenous peoples. Conservation groups, who mostly want more protected areas and fewer people in them, emphasise the emptying of the world's forests and wild places; governments play down the scale of illegal trafficking and the notoriously unhygienic food markets in which wildlife is sometimes sold because it makes them look incompetent; and industries trading animals for the pet and medical trades do not want restrictions, so tend to be secretive. Meanwhile, everyone blames the poorest people for hunting and then selling wild animals.[6]

The net result is that some of the poorest people in the world are routinely blamed for pandemics, and there are very few checks on the health of animals or inspections done at borders. HIV/Aids is widely supposed to have started when an anonymous 'cut' hunter, sometime in the 1940s or earlier, butchered a chimp or some other primate in the Cameroonian rainforest, accidentally infecting himself and then his community.[7]

Some Ebola cases, too, have been linked to the hunting of primates by people living in forests; the SARS pandemic that killed 774 people in 2003 was also widely blamed on catlike mammals called masked civets, which are frequently traded in live animal markets in southern China.[8] Other diseases, such as H5N1 type A influenza, have also been linked to imports of eagles hunted and then imported to Belgium from Thailand.[9]

But blaming hunters and stigmatising wet markets in China and Africa is too easy. HIV/Aids may indeed have been triggered by a Cameroonian hunter, but military campaigns in the forests, prostitution, urbanisation and medical interventions all helped to turn it into the world's most disastrous modern disease. Equally, civet cats in a southern Chinese market are now thought to have been the victims of SARS, rather than the source of the disease; and while some Ebola outbreaks have been linked to indigenous bushmeat hunters, many others appear to have no connection whatsoever.

The deep uncertainty about the origins of so many emerging diseases was seen when Covid-19 appeared, supposedly in the Wuhan wholesale market which had been selling pangolins, bats and other animals capable of being the reservoir of a coronavirus. Spurred on by the Western media, more than 200 conservation groups rushed to condemn hunters and declare the cause of the pandemic to be the high levels of illegal wildlife trade in unhygienic 'wet' markets. The only trouble was that there was no evidence: the disease had not actually started at the Wuhan market and almost certainly had little to do with hunters. As Chinese scientists reported in the *Lancet*, many of the initial cases of Covid-19 had no connection to the market whatsoever. While

Covid-19 may have spread in the market, all the evidence suggests that it is most likely that the disease originated outside and was taken there.

How far hunted animals and wet markets are to blame for disease outbreaks anywhere is highly uncertain. Killing animals in the wild is usually messy but most of the world has long hunted and eaten wild animals without spreading disease. So why should so many diseases be emerging now? The evidence suggests that it's not the hunting or eating of wildlife which is the main problem, so much as whether animals are healthy or not. Bizarrely, conservation may unwittingly be adding to human disease by restricting hunting in certain places.

I came across this in remote Zambia, close to the Malawi border in 2011. I was told of several hundred people living close to the north Luwanga National Park being infected with lethal anthrax poisoning at the same time as hippos were dying of the disease.

Anthrax occurs naturally in the soil here and the disease is endemic, though rare, but that year a long drought had both ruined the staple maize crop local villagers depended on, and left the hippos no grasses to feed on. Because the villages were in a buffer zone where hunting for wildlife was banned, the situation quickly worsened. The hippos began foraging deep into the dry riverbeds for food and water, digging up and swallowing anthrax spores which then killed them, and desperately hungry people then butchered and ate the contaminated dead animals even though they knew the risks. Five people and eighty-five hippos died, and more than 500 people were infected.[10]

I thought back to the Ebola outbreak I had visited in Mayibout 2 in 2004, seven years earlier. The children, I had been told by the chief, had gone into the forest to hunt with dogs, but they had brought back a chimp which they had found dead. I checked whether this had been in the hungry, or lean, season, when food would have been scarce and people hungry enough to eat food they would not normally touch. It was, and moreover the Mayibout 2 outbreak and many others also took place in a drought.[11] So, instead of blaming hunters for the emergence of Ebola, it might have been more accurate to blame hunger, or human-induced climate change. It is equally possible that HIV/Aids emerged by the same route during a drought. Rather than blaming a 'cut' hunter, could it have originated with a troop of hungry soldiers or others finding a dead animal?

* * *

What about wet markets, which are widely blamed in northern countries for the emergence of many zoonotic diseases? Over years of travelling in Latin America, Asia and Africa, I had visited many but while being often shocked by the raw butchery and cruelty that they seemed sometimes to involve, I had come to understand them more as 'farmers' markets' selling fresh, cheap meat especially to poor people. I was also aware that I had never heard reports of diseases starting there.

Perhaps I had got it wrong. Conservation scientists, Western animal welfare groups and some academics trot out the argument that global sickness and pandemics spread from these markets where wild and domestic animals are kept close together, enabling pathogens to jump species. But when challenged they are always reluctant, or unable, to point to specific disease outbreaks starting in markets or with hunters. In theory they are quite correct and the trade in wildlife and wet markets may well be implicated in the spread of some diseases, but that is not proof.

I wanted first-hand, empirical evidence. I started my research in Kisangani, 1,600 or more kilometres up the Congo river, where decades of civil war had cost tens of thousands of human lives and led to vast destruction and political turmoil. The once-great city on the bend in the river in the middle of the second largest tropical forest in the world was shot up and crumbling in the equatorial heat and rains and had become isolated, with no access by road. With its people isolated and now more or less dependent on bushmeat for protein, I imagined Kisangani to be the zoonotic disease capital of the world. Surely here, with nearly all its 500,000 people eating animals hunted in the surrounding forests, there would be zoonotic diseases aplenty.

Kisangani was still pockmarked with bullet holes after three major battles had been fought in its streets only a few years before. It was a vibrant, impoverished frontier town but, ask as I might, no one could tell me of diseases linked to hunting or the eating of wild meat. I checked the hospital and children were indeed dying of diarrhoea and cholera, but no one seemed to be suffering from contaminated bushmeat.

I headed for the Marché Central in the city centre, where it was possible to buy the parts of just about any animal that lived within eighty kilometres of the city – as well as the traps, wires and even home-made guns and bullets that hunters used in the forest. For sale when I visited were live and dead bonobos and chimps, okapi, small antelopes called duikers, monkeys, fruit bats, pangolins, porcupines, warthogs and crocodiles. To my squeamish Western eye, used to seeing meat packed in plastic, it was pretty gruesome, with many clearly distressed animals in cages, blood flowing and butchery taking place in the open. The best-sellers in this world capital of bushmeat were pangolin, duikers, pouched rats and porcupines.

I asked if I could buy some baboon meat. Yes. Elephant? Next week. Gorilla? No. The traders – mostly women – who ran the wildlife part of the market said that hunting had collapsed after Ebola but was now good again and growing, although as the economy improved they were seeing shortages of large animals, because there were too many people demanding them.

'This is the best food, cheap and nutritious. Everyone comes here,' said Marie-Ange Kanza, a boisterous stallholder. But did anyone ever get ill from eating the wild meat? 'No,' she laughed. It was the opposite. 'Fresh meat is safe and good for you. Western meat makes you ill. Just cook it well, *mon ami*!'

On my last night in Kisangani my hosts invited me to eat a smorgasbord of bushmeat from the forest. We started, I think, with duiker (tasty) and moved on to monkey (chewy), bats (sweet), porcupine (mild) and pangolin (good roasted but smelled awful). Everyone in the villages outside Kisangani hunted, I was told, but as the economy picked up after years of conflict, traders were starting to import chicken (bland). Bushmeat was becoming more and more expensive. And, by the way, would I like to invest in a crocodile farm?

Bushmeat has a bad name in the West but across large parts of Central and West Africa, Southeast Asia and Latin America it is a vital source of protein. In remote villages, it is often the only way people can earn money for medicines or to send children to school. Not only are most of the animals hunted small, and prolific breeders, but very few are endangered.[12]

According to Kinshasa-based author and researcher Theodore Trefon, eating certain species has deep symbolic meaning. 'A rich man in Brazzaville who expects his pregnant wife to give birth to a strong boy will provide her with gorilla meat. By eating the meat she appropriates the animal's symbolic strength. At the social level, bushmeat is a frequent item on the table at gatherings with family and friends. It is good etiquette associated with a desire to please, reward, honour, show appreciation or obtain favours,' he said.[13]

No one should know more about the dangers of bushmeat eating and hunting, I thought, than Terese Hart, a legendary American conservationist who went to Zaire (now the Democratic Republic of Congo) as a Peace Corps volunteer in 1974 and, with her anthropologist husband John, set out to explore the vast Ituri forest in eastern Congo with pygmy tribes. She now directs the Lomami National Park, about 300 kilometres south of Kisangani, at the geographic heart of the Congo forest, and runs a major project to protect bonobos. Hunting is banned in the park, but because the local culture is based on it, she allows legal hunters to pass through the protected area with their bushmeat on their way to markets in the biggest nearby town of Kindu.

But for all the years Terese Hart had spent in the forest, and all the conversations she has had with local communities, she said she had not known disease to have been passed to humans from fresh bushmeat.

When we were working in the Ituri Forest in the 1980s and early '90s bushmeat was our main family staple. Mainly duiker meat and only fresh meat. The Mbutii pygmy people in that area did not regularly hunt fruit bats and rarely primates as they were net hunters.

Bushmeat is big here. We have not seen disease linked to it, but that does nothing to make me think that disease is not linked to it; we just have not seen it. Undoubtedly wildlife markets are a possible source of disease. There are some groups like the Mbole (on the northwest side of the Lomami National Park) that eat a lot of fruit bats and string nets through trees to catch them. And shotgun hunters are the most likely to get primates ... So if primates and bats are more likely to be sources there would be groups that would be more at risk than others.[14]

I went back to disease ecologist Thomas Gillespie at Emory University: 'Whenever you have novel interactions with a diverse range of species in one place, whether that is in a natural environment like a forest or an artificially created one like a wet market, you can have a spillover event,' he told me.

These markets bring together a really broad range of animal species from different parts of the forest. They are not eating what they would normally eat in the wild. They are stressed and kept in cages, which lowers their immunity and makes them more susceptible to pathogens. They are butchered, but cutting up an animal and getting its blood on you is a good way to get a pathogen.[15]

* * *

Unable to travel during the Covid-19 lockdown in the UK, I asked a young Nigerian researcher, 'Queenie' Arekpitan, who lives 2,400 kilometres away on the edge of Lagos, Nigeria, to visit West African markets and talk to indigenous hunters and bushmeat buyers about disease.

She went first to the notorious Oluwo market on the eastern edge of Lagos, which is regularly cited by the Western press as a potential zoonotic disease capital.[16] It was disappointing, she said. That day she found monkeys, turtles, tortoises, grasscutters, bush pigs, African giant rats, pangolins, alligators, porcupines, deer, antelopes and civet cats for sale. None were endangered. Other animals usually available included pythons, squirrels and monitor lizards. A big crocodile could be had for $235 and an average-sized python for $13. Crucially, she, too, found no one who thought they had become ill from eating fresh bushmeat:

> The market attracted people from far around from dawn onwards. The biggest customers for pangolins were not Nigerians, but Chinese expatriates. Snakes were being bought mainly by restaurateurs, alligators and crocodiles by Nigerian royalty who wanted them for charms so they could become 'real crocodiles' to their enemies, and the very rich elite who wanted to keep them as pets.
>
> Every Nigerian state has several wildlife markets, with some specialising in snakes, others in crocodiles or leopards, or the animal parts needed by traditional healers. Vulture parts are prized by people who want to see into the future and traditional rulers wanted the by-products of wildlife for aphrodisiacs and ornaments. But outside the exotic animals, the meat was bought by ordinary people.
>
> Many Nigerians will eat an animal if their culture and religion permits it. Usually, consumption peaks during cultural festivals and festive seasons like Christmas and Easter. But young people don't have the taste for bushmeat that their parents had. Nigerians are developing a taste for intercontinental dishes and Western ideas of enjoyment and luxury.[17]

Queenie also conducted a WhatsApp survey of 150 of her family, friends, colleagues and acquaintances. One in ten of them said they had never eaten any wild animal or 'weird' meat. The rest had tried at least one of a long list that included monkeys, mamba, python and cobras, bush dogs, gorillas, bats and turtles. 'In general, people in villages ate more bushmeat, and young urbanites, while still enjoying bushmeat, were losing their parents' taste for it,' she said. Again, none were put off because they had become ill.

But was Lagos representative? I also asked Queenie to find and talk to hunters about disease. In a series of interviews with people who had spent decades trapping and butchering animals, she found no one who had ever heard of diseases being passed from animals to humans. They were all poor, mostly killing their prey in the forest, but none took special health precautions. Instead, they all took charms, special herbs and objects with them to protect themselves from evil. They were all convinced after years of hunting all kinds of animal in all regions that wild animals were healthy.

Kolawoje Ajayi was typical. A middle-aged man from Mowe in Ogun State, he had hunted snakes, antelopes and monkeys for decades and learned to treat the forests with respect. 'When you kill some dangerous animals you make sure you perform some sacrifices and rituals to absolve you of your actions,' he said. 'Eating well-cooked meat is the key to staying well. If you cook it properly you can cook away any disease.' He believed that the bats he had heard were linked to Covid-19 and Ebola had not been not properly roasted. 'The people who get diseases are the ones, like in the abattoirs, who eat raw animal flesh. Not hunters.'

Kehinde, who sold bushmeat in Benin City, said that the diseases to beware of affected the hunter rather than the wider community. Hunters, he said, had peculiar rules to follow passed down by families, like to avoid the livers of any four-legged wild animals, and never to eat a lion's kidney (indeed, if a fly touched a lion's kidney and then touched you, it would lead to instant death, he insisted). 'When you slaughter a boar, do not mention anyone's name. If you do, the spirit of the animal will attack that person. If that doesn't happen, on your next hunt, you'll be attacked yourself by a boar.'

Samuel Osawaru used dogs to hunt antelopes, deer, porcupines, monkeys and the occasional baboon. He was less concerned with disease than with the dwarves who lived in the forests, who appeared like shadows and which you could smell from far away. 'There are "diabolical things" in the forest,' he said. 'Animals sometimes change to humans and vice versa.'

So, I asked John Fa, coordinator of the Bushmeat Research Initiative at the UN's Center for International Forestry (CIFOR), who had spent many years researching diet and disease in central Africa, whether it should be banned. 'It is important not to throw the baby out with the bathwater,' he said. 'Wild meat plays an important role in the nutrition of large populations of humans, accounting for up to 50 per cent of the protein intake of people in central Africa. You can't just say to people: "You can't do it any more."'

Wildlife hunting bans mostly fail, said Stephanie Brittain, who spent five years in Cameroon researching bushmeat consumption and now works with Oxford University's Interdisciplinary Centre for Conservation Science. After the 2013–16 Ebola outbreak in West Africa, she says, bans were brought in by several countries but could not be policed. The result was an increase in hunting for wild meat.[18] 'There [is] no conclusive evidence that banning the wildlife trade will prevent the emergence of zoonotic diseases in the future. Bans can drive trade underground, resulting in illegal markets with lower hygiene regulation and increased risk of disease,' she told me.

Delia Grace, programme leader for food safety and zoonoses at the International Livestock Research Institute in Nairobi, Kenya, put the debate into perspective. 'Wet markets are basically fresh food markets. In the UK we like farmers' markets with fresh corn-fed chickens, farm-sourced meats and nice-looking sausages. That's basically a wet market, though in a different cultural context. They are essential to bring fresh food to urban populations, and provide for the food security of millions of people. They do need to be regulated and controlled. But they should not be blanket banned, as that is not sensitive to the needs of their clients who depend on them.'[19]

Conservationists still argue strongly for market closures but anyone with first-hand knowledge of zoonotic diseases, at least in Africa, is more cautious. Eric Fèvre, chair of veterinary services and infectious diseases at the University of Liverpool, and Cecilia

Tacoli, researcher in the human settlements research group at the International Institute for Environment and Development (IIED), together argued that 'rather than pointing the finger at wet markets, we should look at the burgeoning trade in wild animals. It is wild animals rather than farmed animals that are the natural hosts of many viruses. But … evidence shows the link between informal markets and disease is not always clear-cut.'[20]

Yvan, a villager living near the Dja biosphere reserve in Cameroon, summed up the attitude of many African communities on learning that Covid-19 might have started in wild meat: 'Why is it that before, even during our ancestors' era, this disease did not catch us? I think that white people are lying to us. They produce things and now it is having impacts on us black people.'[21]

I put my findings to Thomas Gillespie and suggested that the loud calls at the start of the Covid-19 pandemic to ban markets and to stop hunting on health grounds may have been hasty. 'I have tensions at times with conservationists pushing this as a critical issue. They are a risk, but nowhere as great as the clearing of forests and the intensive farming of animals,' he said.

* * *

Epidemics always seem to strike unexpectedly, and there was consternation in June 2003 when ninety people across the states of Illinois, Indiana and New Jersey were found to have contracted human Mpox.[22] This disease had been identified for the first time in the Democratic Republic of Congo only in 1970 and since then had been limited to sporadic outbreaks in remote West African villages, occasionally jumping to Europe. Some monkeys and a few rabbits and rats were known to harbour the virus but only occasionally had it been known to spread from human to human. In 2022 cases started appearing in the UK, the Netherlands and more than a dozen other countries, but in 2003 it was quite unknown in Wisconsin.

How did a rainforest disease rarely seen in people get to the US Midwest, where cows and deer nearly outnumber people? In an extraordinary piece of detective work, the outbreak was traced back to a three-year-old girl who had been scratched by a small native American rodent, misleadingly called a prairie dog, that her parents had bought for her from the local meat inspector at a summer 'swap party', or street market.[23] This prairie dog, it emerged, had shared a ride to Wisconsin with several hundred small mammals, including squirrels, dormice and some caged Gambian giant rats, all recently imported from Ghana by a pet trader. One of the giant rats in the consignment from Africa had been infected with Mpox and passed it to the prairie dog.

In the last thirty years there has been an explosion in the number of pets and companion animals people keep, to the point where more than half of all households in the US, UK, Australia and much of the EU include at least one animal. Where it used to be common to keep a dog or a cat, it is common now for people to have snakes, rats, hamsters, guinea pigs, hedgehogs, rodents, bearded dragons, chinchillas, birds, turtles and ferrets.[24] Exotic pet websites abound, offering everything from pocket monkeys ($6,900) and warthogs ($6,000) to camels ($12,500), even wolves.

But while pets may be great for human fitness, stress and mental health, they regularly infect people with their pathogens. Mostly this is no problem, because our immune systems have adapted, but the US government have registered more than 100 often lurid diseases that can be passed from pets and their food to humans,[25] and every year records many outbreaks of salmonella and other serious diseases.

Increasingly, says Bruno Chomel, emerging disease epidemiologist at the University of California, Davis, we may be risking catching new diseases. 'Affluence and fashion are now leading to larger pet and companion animal populations. The exponential growth of human population is leading to more incursions in natural habitats and exposure to pathogens naturally infecting wildlife.[26] Our domesticated animals then can be a relay for some of these pathogens.'[27]

Exotic pets and companion animals have become so numerous that they now pose a real risk to human health. Birds, reptiles and rodents carry salmonella, dogs can pass rabies to humans, cats pass

roundworm and cat scratch disease to humans and African pygmy
hedgehogs or chinchillas spread nervous diseases. 'So far there have
been no major epidemics or pandemics starting in the home. But
there have been large outbreaks with hundreds of human cases of
psittacosis, salmonella, tularemia, lymphocytic choriomeningitis
virus and worse from reptiles, rodents and exotic birds or pigeons,'
says Chomel.[28]

Petting farms and zoos, as well as circuses and ecotourism, have
all been linked to outbreaks of salmonellosis and infectious diseases.
Elephant handlers, children and farm workers are contracting
diseases like meningitis, Q fever and chagas. 'In some Middle
East countries, it has become trendy to have exotic carnivores as
pets. Movies such as *Jurassic Park* have led to an increase in the
ownership of reptiles like iguanas in lieu of dinosaurs and can easily
spread salmonella. Most reptiles are natural carriers of Salmonella
bacteria,' he writes in an email. Counter-intuitively, in a world
where nature is said to be in steep decline and large animals are
becoming rare, we have never been closer to other species.

* * *

Instead of stigmatising hunters and demanding a stop to the legal
bushmeat trade, there is a growing realisation that zoonotic disease
in China and South Asia may be linked to the many semi-legal,
unregulated and intensive wildlife farms that have sprouted in the
last forty years and send their food to urban markets like Wuhan.
Here large numbers of captive wild animals are selectively bred
for their meat and fur, and for medicine. There may be little or
no monitoring of the conditions they are kept in, and not much
is known about the diseases that may be circulating, but Hong
Kong City University vet Ioannis Magouras, lead author of a 2020
international study, says that avian flu is known to have emerged
in ostrich farms in South Africa, rabies in kudu farms and SARS-
Cov-2 in mink farms in the Netherlands.

From just a handful of these wild animal farms forty years ago,
there are now tens of thousands in Vietnam, China, Laos, Cambodia
and Thailand. One UN census of just twelve provinces in Vietnam

found over 4,000 working farms breeding more than 1.5 million animals from 185 different species, including porcupines, bats, snakes, turtles, civets, primates and wild boar. Similar numbers are thought to have opened in Laos, Cambodia and China. Not all the animals came directly from nature but most had direct contact with wild animals. Mortalities were high and few, it was said, had any veterinary support.[29]

These farms boomed from the 1980s after China actively promoted the mass farming and trading of wildlife as a way to bring rural populations out of poverty when the country was industrialising. Thousands were set up by provinces and helped the local governments meet ambitious goals of closing the rural–urban divide. By 2016, says Peter Daszak, one of the WHO team investigating the source of Covid-19, they employed 14 million people and it was a $70 billion success story.

The WHO, having started its investigation into the source of Covid-19 suspecting it was the Wuhan market, now thinks one of these farms may have been responsible. Why else, Daszak asked the world's press at the end of its investigation in March 2021, did the authorities declare that they were going to stop the farming of wildlife for food and send out instructions to the farmers about how to safely dispose of the animals – to bury, kill or burn them – in a way that didn't spread disease?[30]

'Why would the government do this?' he asked rhetorically. In an interview with NPR and others in March 2021 he told how wildlife farms were breeding animals like civet cats and pangolins known to carry coronaviruses, and were trading them with vendors at the Huanan Seafood Wholesale Market in Wuhan. The wildlife farms, rather than hunters, provided a perfect conduit between a coronavirus-infected bat in Yunnan (or neighbouring Myanmar) and a Wuhan animal market, he said.[31]

'China closes that pathway down for a reason,' he continued. 'The reason was, back in February 2020, they believed this was the most likely pathway [for the coronavirus to spread to Wuhan]. And when the WHO report comes out … we believe it's the most likely pathway, too.'[32]

10

FURTHER, FASTER

Wildlife tourists flock to the Meru National Park in the foothills of Mount Kenya. This is where the 1960s big-budget film *Born Free* was set and where Elsa the lioness and her cubs famously lived. But very few people who go there ever pause at the huge bronze figure of a Cape buffalo which stands guard on a plinth by the main gate. Elephants and giraffes sometimes approach the statue thinking it is alive, but these days it is barely remarked on that this is where one of the world's most devastating and ancient animal diseases officially ended its journey after travelling the world for centuries.

It was here at Meru in 2002 that the very last outbreak of rinderpest, or cattle plague, was ended and an horrendous chapter in human and animal history could be declared over. The disease, which probably originated in the steppes of Mongolia, emerging when people first started to domesticate cattle 10,000 or more years ago, had weakened civilisations for millennia, led to many human famines and changed the physical face of continents.

Spread by traders and by Genghis Khan and successive armies on their campaigns, it had, since the eighteenth century, swept many times through Europe, killing hundreds of millions of cattle and other animals in Germany, France and Britain. It was said to have preceded the fall of Rome, the conquest of Christian Europe by Charlemagne and the French Revolution. Remarkably, it had never caught hold in sub-Saharan Africa.

So when, in November 1888, it arrived in the Red Sea port of Massawa in what is now Eritrea, in a small herd of Asian grey steppe oxen brought by Italian soldiers, it was unopposed and unknown. Within a decade, Africa – a continent three times the size of Europe – had been socially and ecologically ravaged by what has become known as the Great African Pandemic.

Possibly the infected cattle were known to be diseased and their introduction to Africa was a deliberate ploy by the Italian colonial army to overcome an enemy, but it could just as well have been an accident. Either way, within months of the animals' arrival, hundreds and then thousands of local cattle and wild animals which had no resistance to the deadly virus were dropping dead, wracked with fevers and diarrhoea.

Rinderpest was transmitted both by contact between animals and through drinking water. It did not affect people directly, but remains a terrible warning of how an animal disease can decimate human lives and create centuries of social and economic chaos. On a continent where as many as half the people at the time were semi-nomadic pastoralists and nearly everyone depended on cattle for their health, wealth and culture, it was utterly savage.

Cattle were not just prized, but were life itself for Africa's many great tribes like the Fulani, Dinka, Maasai and Samburu. Cows conferred power and influence, were used as currency, praised and sung to, and anything that harmed them was liable to undermine power structures and ravage the livelihoods of communities.

The devastation was probably even greater than that caused by the pulses of bubonic plague that coursed through Europe in the Middle Ages. Following ox trails, caravan and migratory animal routes, it spread south through what is now Tanzania, Mozambique, the Democratic Republic of Congo and Botswana to reach South Africa in 1897. Heading west across the Sahel via Chad, Nigeria and Ghana, rinderpest took five years to reach the Atlantic, along the way igniting wars, famine and social upheaval.[1] Not only did it kill 90 per cent or more of the cattle and wildlife wherever it went, it led to the deaths by starvation of millions of people and untold numbers of both wild and domestic animals, and changed the fauna and flora of Africa south of the Sahara completely.[2]

Rinderpest decimated upwards of forty species, including sheep, goats, wildebeest and antelopes. Carcasses were left on the land, encouraging human diseases like smallpox, typhus, cholera and influenza, and lands became graveyards. Farmers had no draught animals to plough their fields and no dung for fertiliser, so crops failed. Tribal structures were weakened, allowing colonial powers to move in unopposed, and parents are said to have sold their children to slave masters. With food scarce, large areas became depopulated.

Even as rinderpest was being brought under control and the last case had been detected, I visited Richard Pankhurst, the great historian of Ethiopia, at his home in Addis Ababa. I asked how important rinderpest had been. He put it on a par with colonialism. 'It physically and socially changed the continent completely. The Africa you see today is not the Africa that existed before the disease.'[3]

David Morens, a medical historian and infectious disease expert at the US National Institutes of Health, picks up the story:

Desperate for food ... people abandoned their farms and villages to forage, consuming leaves and roots, picking through animal dung for undigested seeds, and eating the rotting corpses of horses, dogs, hyenas, jackals, and vultures. Some turned to cannibalism. Parents sold their children into slavery in the hope that slave masters would save the childrens' lives by feeding them. Others committed suicide and murder. Smallpox epidemics broke out. Starving people fell and died in the forests, along roadsides, and around churches. Lions, leopards, and jackals began to attack and kill people in broad daylight.[4]

Morens and others have argued that rinderpest was even the ultimate cause of the second Matabele War in 1896. Such was the reduction in the numbers of food animals and dairy cattle and the resultant hunger and health problems that the Matabele and other peoples in what is now Zimbabwe revolted. In some parts of East Africa death rates from hunger among tribal peoples are estimated to have reached one half to two-thirds of the population.[5]

But environment writer Fred Pearce and others contend that rinderpest may also have sparked a very important longer-term ecological revolution which utterly changed the fortunes and politics of large parts of the continent, altering ecosystems, bringing disease, helping colonists seize land and laying the foundations for modern Africa. According to Pearce, the seemingly pristine, wild Africa so often portrayed on modern film and TV as full of wildlife was largely formed in the nineteenth century by a tiny, invading alien pathogen.[6]

His argument is rooted in common sense.[7] Before it arrived in Africa, the great wandering plant-eating herds of buffalo, wildebeest and cattle historically kept by pastoralists grazed the bush and kept down the dreaded tsetse fly, a small biting insect which transmits a disease called trypanosomiasis, or sleeping sickness, to both humans and cattle. But, he says, with cattle, buffalo, antelope, elan, giraffe, goats and nearly all cloven-hoofed animals killed by rinderpest, a new landscape of thorn bush and trees ideal for tsetse flies to breed in quickly grew across vast areas.

The absence of grazing animals allowed the fly to colonise old pasturelands rapidly and expand its range into areas which it had never known before, and, despite countless attempts to eradicate it, it has never been exterminated since. In the wake of rinderpest successive epidemics of sleeping sickness killed many millions of people.

Just as waves of human and animal disease changed the Americas in the wake of colonisation and slavery, so the effects of rinderpest have cascaded down the years in Africa. Sleeping sickness has been now more or less confined to western and central Africa but the damage done in the nineteenth century lingers. When Europeans came to Africa, they found nations weak from population decline, hunger and disease caused by both rinderpest and the tsetse fly. Vast areas of land which once provided food and wealth for people but which were then infested by the fly or depopulated by rinderpest are now fenced off, occupied by foreign-owned game reserves and national parks which favour wild animals over people or are still uninhabitable by humans or their cattle.

* * *

Rinderpest travelled through Africa at the walking pace of a man or a herd of cattle on the move – a few kilometres a day. By comparison, the far more virulent 1918 Spanish flu virus, which possibly killed one in ten people it infected, took two years to sweep the world, travelling mostly by boat. Covid-19, by contrast, spread to nearly every country in the world within a few weeks after a cluster of cases of 'a pneumonia of unknown origin' emerged in a Wuhan seafood market in December 2019.

Covid-19 was super-spread by plane. Within days it had reached Japan, France and twenty-five other countries. By mid-February 2020 it was in thirty-seven more countries and by May 2020 it had infected people in every country and territory of the world, apart from Turkmenistan, North Korea and five Pacific islands. It was by no means the deadliest of diseases, but thanks to tourism and trade it was by far the furthest – and fastest – global pandemic in recorded history.

The difference in the speed at which rinderpest, Spanish flu and Covid-19 spread round the world comes down simply to technology. In 1918 railways and steamships rather than aeroplanes connected the world. It took fourteen days or more to cross the Atlantic, and two months at least to go to Australia from Europe by steamship. In 2020, it took hours. In 1914 the cartographer John G. Bartholomew published a map showing how long it would take a traveller – or a pathogen he or she might carry – to get between different points. From London to New York was five to ten days, but to most of Africa and Australia it was six weeks. There were steam trains and ships but they were few and far between.[8]

Today, I can leave London feeling unwell on a night flight to Nairobi and pass an illness to a remote Malawian villager twelve hours later. We – and that includes our microbes – are now all just a few hours' flight away from places that in the past would have taken months or years to travel to by land or sea. Travellers have always spread disease but nowadays they can bring a disease halfway across the world almost before they know they are sick.

The larger the world population and the more crowded humanity has become, the more we travel and the more we accelerate the speed at which diseases emerge and spread. Past pandemics were mostly spread by traders, pilgrims or soldiers. In a rural and isolated world with fewer people there were far fewer interactions between people and animals. Increased mobility, more than any evolution of microbes today, drives pandemics.

The 1889 influenza travelled from Asia to Europe along newly built railroad lines and was then carried along old shipping routes. The 1957 flu pandemic was also spread by ships, but eleven years later, the 1968 pandemic, which may have killed 4 million people as it travelled round the world, became the first to be predominantly spread by commercial aviation.

Trade, war and colonialism, above all, have changed the geography of disease. Twelfth-century European crusaders to the Holy Land brought back leprosy from the Middle East; bubonic plague was carried back and forth along the Silk Road from China to Europe; the slave trade took smallpox and influenza to the Americas and by the nineteenth century British, German, French and Spanish colonisers were not just taking the resources of Africa, Latin America and Asia, but bringing diseases such as cholera, measles, gonorrhoea, typhoid and plague.

Stowaway rats are said to have brought the Black Death from Asia in the twelve boats which docked at the Sicilian port of Messina in 1347. Columbus took measles, chickenpox and possibly smallpox to the New World and traders brought by ship the rats which carried the bacteria that led to the Plague of Justinian (AD 541–42), which devastated the Byzantine Empire. The first cholera epidemic, thought to have started in India with

British colonials, was spread across the world by the British navy. It travelled along the West African coast by boat and into the interior along rivers.[9]

How impossible it is to stop a microorganism hitching a ride on a boat or a train can be seen in the vain attempts of countries to keep cholera at bay in the nineteenth century. The death march from the east of this horrifying, waterborne disease, which can dehydrate and shrivel someone in a day, was tracked month by month by governments for five years in the 1820s.

As it travelled from Bengal across Asia and then slowly through Western Europe to the Baltic seaports, it was observed to move no faster than coaches and ships, slowing down in the winter when people travelled less, and picking up speed again in the summer as trade increased. It paused for nearly a year when it reached the Baltic in 1831, seemingly giving the new British government under Lord Grey time to prepare their defences. With admirable prescience, hundreds of ships loaded with flax, hemp and other goods were quarantined for weeks off the northeast coast of England.

For a few months in the summer of 1831 it looked as if cholera would remain in mainland Europe. But as has been seen with Covid-19, pathogens are anything but predictable. Sailors from a Russian tar ferry are said to have carried the disease ashore at Sunderland in northeast England, but medical historian Ethne Barnes suggests that it was not the sailors who carried it but the cholera-infected bilge waters of their quarantined ships, which spread the disease by contaminating the fish and shellfish that were widely eaten by local people. 'The quarantine to prevent cholera turned into a guarantee of the disease,' she wrote in 2005.[10] The disease soon spread north to Scotland and south to London, probably on boats carrying coal. Eventually the 1831 epidemic killed an estimated 52,000 people in Britain.

Fifty-six years after cholera landed in Sunderland at the height of European imperialism, Dr Richard Thorne Thorne, the vice-president of the British Medical Association, could write that seaborne disease seemed 'unstoppable' and was likely to ruin

Europe. 'It is from sea-borne cholera that Europe now runs the greatest risk: Vessel after vessel, troopship, mail steamer and merchantman pass it [cholera] on as it were in one continuous line from the east to ports. A desperate struggle has been made to uphold the [quarantine] system but the system is altogether elusive,' he reported in 1887 in the *British Medical Journal*.[11]

* * *

Each of the world's first six great cholera pandemics was spread by people travelling on water. As befits a waterborne disease, the seventh, which is still going on and had infected people in thirty-four countries by 2017, started on the Indonesian island of Sulawesi in 1961.[12] In the sixty years since it has steadily spread through the slums of Asia and Africa.[13] In 2000 a team of Smithsonian Institution researchers tested fifteen ships arriving in Chesapeake Bay on the East Coast of North America and found that a litre of ballast water contained around 830 million bacteria and 7,400 million viruses.[14] *Vibrio cholerae*, the bacterium that causes cholera, was detected in the ballast plankton of all fifteen of them. More recent research suggests that genes for antimicrobial resistance are also spreading among microbes in ballast water,[15] and that infected water from cruise liners is responsible for the devastating stony coral tissue loss disease now spreading throughout the Mayan reef system and the Caribbean.[16]

The chances of these microorganisms directly infecting humans is next to impossible, but they are known to affect fisheries and in this way to reach humans. In the case of Chancay, it is likely that some *Vibrio cholerae* bacteria were ingested by shellfish which was then eaten raw, kicking off the devastating 1992 Latin American cholera epidemic.[17]

Within a few weeks cholera had spread 2,000 kilometres up and down the Pacific coast ports on intercontinental ships, soon transferring to seafood and water to reach the mountains and forests of Bolivia, Ecuador, Argentina, Colombia and Brazil. By the end of 1992 more than 1 million of Latin America's poorest people had been infected and 11,000 had died. It would have been far more but for the prompt action of the authorities.[18]

A travelling virus may also cause vast economic damage. SARS cost billions of dollars in 2003 by cutting international travel by 50 to 70 per cent. Growth of the Chinese GDP fell. The Covid-19 coronavirus has cost trillions.

* * *

While air travel may have spread Covid-19 further and faster than ever before, cruise ships are well-known incubators and carriers of Legionnaires' disease, hepatitis A, flu and stomach bugs. Analysis of 53 cruise ships which left the world's ports between mid-January and March 2020 suggests that all but two had outbreaks of Covid-19, and nearly 3,000 people were confirmed to have been infected on board.[19]

It was hardly surprising. When travellers from many regions and multicultural crews are brought together in crowded, enclosed environments, person-to-person, diseases will inevitably thrive. In 2019 the *Oasis of the Seas*, at the time the world's largest cruise ship, had to return to Florida from a Caribbean cruise when 561 out of 6,285 passengers fell ill with a norovirus.[20] 'As people sleep, eat and socialise in a tight space such as a cruise ship, viruses and bacteria can move even faster,' commented the US Centers of Disease Control and Prevention (CDC).[21]

Ships, indeed, have been super-spreaders. One hundred years ago, ships spread what became known as the Spanish flu to and from troops fighting in Europe. The official report from 29 September 1918 by the chief medical officer of USS *Leviathan*, the biggest ship in the world at the time, gives a vivid account of one of the grimmest voyages any ship may ever have made. In fatally overcrowded conditions the flu virus was spread easily between people and went on to infect and kill thousands more in France.[22]

'The ship was packed, conditions were such that the influenza bacillus could breed and multiply with extraordinary swiftness. There are no means of knowing the actual number of sick at any one time but it is estimated that 700 cases developed by the night of September 30. They were brought to the sick bay from all parts of the ship in a continuous stream only to be turned away because all the beds were occupied. Each succeeding day was a nightmare of weariness and anxiety,' the record states.

The *Leviathan* became known as the 'death ship': 'It is the opinion of myself and the other medical officers attached to the ship that there were fully 2,000 cases of influenza on board … Records were impossible, and even identification of patients was extremely difficult … many were either delirious or too ill to know their own names,' the report states. 'It was pitiful to see men toppling over dead at your feet. It was like some invisible hand reaching out and suddenly taking them away.'[23] Hundreds died on board the *Leviathan* and a further 123 who travelled on her died within days of landing at Brest in France. Of the 9,100 troops and crew aboard, one in four are known to have contracted the disease and many are likely to have passed it on to other soldiers.

The *Leviathan*'s grim voyages to and from France were not remotely comparable to those of the *Diamond Princess* or the *Ruby Princess*, two of the world's largest and most luxurious cruise liners, which within a week of each other in early 2020 took thousands of international holidaymakers and their pathogens on expensive escapes. The *Diamond Princess* left Yokohama on 20 January for a fourteen-day round trip of Southeast Asia. Few of the 2,666 passengers and 1,045 crew paid much attention when people started coughing. By the time the liner returned on 1 March, more than 712 people were infected with Covid-19 and fourteen people from Japan, the UK, Canada and elsewhere had died. One week later, the *Ruby Princess*, with a similar quota of elderly holidaymakers and families, left Sydney, Australia, to circumnavigate New Zealand. They never got there. By Day 10 the *Ruby Princess*'s cruise had become a nightmare for the ship's sole doctor, who reported to management that dozens of people were being taken ill and some were developing fevers.

On Day 11 an elderly woman died and the ship was ordered to cut the voyage short and return to Sydney. When the *Ruby Princess* finally docked, 110 people on board were seriously sick and seventeen had a fever. Inexplicably, the passengers were then allowed to leave the ship and disperse around Australia, taking Covid-19 with them. In the following weeks, more than 700 passengers and 202 crew tested positive and twenty-two people died, a remarkably similar percentage of infections and deaths to those on both the *Leviathan* in 1918 and the *Diamond Princess*. The *Leviathan* in 1918 had been dubbed the 'charnel ship'; a hundred years later the two cruise liners were being called 'death traps'.

* * *

Aviation is now the great super-spreader of pandemics. The Americans found this out in 2017 when a Liberian, Thomas Duncan, walked into a Dallas hospital complaining of stomach aches and was sent home with a few pills. Three days later, the man who had flown from Monrovia to Dallas via Brussels and Washington without showing any symptoms started vomiting and returned to the hospital begging for help. After one week his organs were collapsing. The first American case of Ebola miraculously travelled no further. In only slightly different circumstances, Duncan could have passed one of the world's most feared diseases to dozens of people in four large cities on three continents in just two days. The consequences are unimaginable.

Not only are there more outbreaks of infectious diseases to be spread to far more people than there were only a hundred years ago, but diseases are becoming globalised as human populations become more closely connected by trade, traffic and tourism. In 2019 health ecologist Serge Morand from French Agricultural research centre CNRS-CIRAD, and Bruno Walther from the National Sun Yat-Sen University in Taiwan, analysed data from the World Bank and Gideon, a global disease database which tracks the outbreaks of over 350 diseases in 220 countries. They wanted to see if there was a link between the growth of international travel and the increase in the number of disease outbreaks since the Second World War.

The answer was categorically yes. By any measure, the world has been on the move as never before in the past seventy years.

Since 1945 the number of cars has increased six times to 1.2 billion, the number of international tourists has jumped from around 25 million a year to over 1.4 billion, and the amount of trade carried by sea has increased from 0.5 to 11 billion megatons a year. In that time there have been 17,494 confirmed disease outbreaks in 221 countries and territories. 'Before 1962, a disease outbreak usually remained confined to one or a few closely connected countries; thereafter, disease outbreaks have become increasingly pandemic in their nature,' say Morand and Walther, who added: 'One cost of increased global mobility (which is currently tightly linked to economic growth and globalization) … is the increased risk of disease outbreaks and their faster and wider spread.'[24]

* * *

Today disease can be a sheer numbers game. In the 1970s, according to World Bank and industry data, there were around 330 million air passengers a year and around 500 million tonnes of freight was transported by sea. By 2019 there were nearly 200,000 flights a day from the world's airports, and a fleet of 60,000 or more cargo ships was at sea at any one time. Both air and sea traffic had grown exponentially, more than 1,200 per cent in just one generation.[25]

Not only has the number of disease outbreaks reported annually by governments more than tripled since the 1980s, but so has the number of countries affected by any disease outbreak. What is more, the countries with the most outbreaks have been the countries which are the most served by major air hubs.[26]

According to Morand and Walther, the US, which has the most international air passenger traffic, has had 1,824 disease outbreaks since the 1940s, far more than any other country. It is followed by the UK (927), India (653), Canada (565), Japan (547), Australia (467) and China (432).[27] When Morand and colleagues interrogated the databases more deeply, they found that clusters of disease outbreaks have increasingly become connected with other clusters. Before 1962, an outbreak usually remained confined to one or just a few closely connected countries; now they are becoming increasingly pandemic, spreading quickly to many countries.

They concluded that there has been a great acceleration of infectious disease risks in the last sixty to seventy years. Global connectivity due to air traffic allows an outbreak to rapidly spread across several national and continental borders very quickly. In short, the cost of increased global mobility is the increased risk of disease outbreaks.

The role of both aviation and shipping was clearly seen in at least the first months of the Covid-19 pandemic. The countries that were most impacted first were the ones like the UK and the US, where large airport hubs allowed people and goods to travel most easily. Milan, Paris, Brussels, Frankfurt and London in Europe and New York in the US created the major exchanges for the virus to grow. Winter tourist hotspots like Spain in the northern hemisphere, as well as Alpine and Rocky Mountain ski resorts, were also badly affected. In a second wave of infections, business people and tourists travelling from primary centres in Europe and China transported the disease to Africa and Latin America.

Today increased global mobility is one of the great drivers of modern pandemics. The aviation industry confidently expects the amount of freight carried by air to double and the numbers of international tourists to increase by 400 million within fifteen years. Put simply, if that happens, we can expect far more pandemics.[28]

* * *

Covid-19 was not the first disease to be spread primarily by aviation. In an eerie foretaste of 2020, another coronavirus disease also linked to wild animals, and that also started in Guangdong province in southern China, spread like a cancer, slowly at first, then metastasising to other countries by air within a few months. SARS, or South Asian respiratory syndrome, showed once again how hard it is to stop any disease spreading in a crowded, globalised, interconnected world and how luck, as much as anything, plays a role in disease transmission. But it also showed how quick-thinking authorities can contain or slow a pandemic even as it is taking to the air and sea.[29]

As with so many modern diseases, from the start SARS was linked to meat. Of the first seven patients to be admitted to the Sun Yat-Sen Memorial Hospital in Guangzhou in 2002, several were restaurant chefs and one had in the previous weeks cooked snake, domestic cat and chicken for his family. Four had died. Of the people they affected, aside from health workers, many were wild food handlers, including a snake seller.

For several weeks there were only small, sporadic outbreaks. By Christmas, rumours were rife that a fatal disease was circulating in the province. The first 'super-spreader' was probably Zhou Zuofen, a fish seller from Guangzhou, who went to hospital on 31 January 2002. He died within a week, but before he did, he is said to have infected thirty medical staff at the hospital, who in turn spread it to two other hospitals.

As with Covid-19, it was frontline health workers who, tragically, suffered most. One of the doctors in Guangzhou was a respiratory doctor, Liu Jianiun, who on 21 February took the three-hour bus ride to Hong Kong to see family and attend a wedding. That evening the 64-year-old professor booked room 911 on the ninth floor of the large Metropole hotel in the Kowloon area of the city.

At some point Liu probably sneezed or coughed, possibly in or close to a hotel lift. Somehow, he transmitted the disease to sixteen others in the hotel, including eight people on his floor. The next morning, Liu – by now worried about his deteriorating health – walked the five blocks from the hotel to Kwong Wah Hospital, where doctors took no chances and put him straight into an isolation ward. Even though the hospital workers wore masks, gloves and gowns, one doctor and five nurses were infected.

Until this point the still-unnamed disease had remained more or less local and contained. But it then hitched a ride on a plane with tourists and business people. Of the eight people infected on Liu's hotel floor, at least four took it around the globe within days. An elderly woman, Sui-Chu Kwan, travelled to Toronto, where it killed her and a further forty-two people. A businessman took it to Taiwan, where 181 people died and 668 others were infected, and a woman, Esther Mok, flew to Singapore, where 238 people were infected and thirty-three died.

The fourth was Johnny Chen, a Chinese American living in Shanghai who like Zhou Zuofen was staying overnight at the Metropole, but who flew the next day to Hanoi in Vietnam. There he fell ill and checked in to the Hanoi French Hospital, thinking he had the flu. There he infected at least forty-five people, including an anaesthetist who was examined on 5 March by Carlo Urbani, a young Italian microbiologist working with the World Health Organization.

Urbani is a true hero. His quick thinking alerted the world and certainly slowed the spread of SARS throughout much of Southeast Asia. Seeing how other hospital staff were becoming ill, he alone realised that Chen was suffering from a new and dangerous contagious disease. He immediately warned the WHO headquarters in Geneva, Switzerland, and the Vietnamese government. The disease was officially named SARS. Two weeks later, on a flight to Bangkok to attend a conference on childhood parasites, Urbani himself took ill. He had contracted SARS from one of his patients in Hanoi and died after eighteen days in intensive care.

By then, the virus was nearly out of control, with outbreaks popping up all over Asia, triggering panic and fear. Armed guards patrolled hospitals, passengers suspected of having the disease were hauled off planes, businesses and schools were closed. Twenty-three other guests from the Metropole developed SARS and, perhaps via rats or cockroaches, the virus got into the drains and plumbing system of a dense cluster of apartment blocks called Amoy Gardens, where it infected 320 people and killed thirty-three. In the end it travelled by plane to twenty-nine countries, infected more than 8,000 people and killed 774, a mortality rate of almost 10 per cent. If Covid-19 had been as lethal, it would have killed at least 2.5 million people within the first six months, instead of 800,000.

I called Jamie Bartram, the former head of water, sanitation, hygiene and health at the WHO. 'The world really dodged a bullet with SARS, and because the experience was not that bad for large swathes of the world, we failed to learn our lessons from it. It was an alarm call we all slept through. It shows how fragile we are and how exposed people can be to virulent pandemic disease.'[30]

For most of history, says Mary E. Wilson, professor of global health at Harvard University, human populations were relatively isolated and it has only been in recent centuries that there has been extensive contact between the flora and fauna of the Old and New Worlds. Wilson, who has studied the linked movements of human and plant pathogens across the world for nearly fifty years, says that by the end of the fifteenth century, measles, influenza, mumps, smallpox, tuberculosis and other infections had all become common in Europe thanks to increasing travel.

Explorers from the crowded urban centres of Europe brought infectious diseases to the New World, where isolated populations had evolved from a relatively small gene pool and had no previous experience with many infections. The first epidemics following the arrival of Europeans were often the most severe. By 1518 or 1519 smallpox appeared in Santo Domingo, now the capital of the Dominican Republic, where it killed possibly half the population and spread to other areas of the Caribbean and the Americas. The population of central Mexico is estimated to have dropped by one-third in the single decade following first contact with the Europeans.

Wilson reminds us that diseases emerge when we travel or migrate. 'We carry with us our microbes and biological life and we inevitably change the environments we pass through. People change the environment in many ways when they travel or migrate – they plant, clear land, build, and consume. Travel leads to the emergence of disease if it changes an ecosystem.'[31]

11

BEWARE THE BIRDS

On the evening of 7 August 2018, a KLM charter flight left Amsterdam in Europe, landing eleven hours later at Kilimanjaro airport in northern Tanzania. The young travellers were nodded past customs officials and driven eighty kilometres to their new home. These were no wealthy gap-year students eager to climb Africa's nearby highest peak or tourists paying top dollar to watch lions in the Serengeti National Park, but a flock of elite 'super-chickens'. The destination of these 2,320 Cobb 500 cockerels and 17,208 hens was a 200-hectare megafarm being built on the windy plain leading to the foothills of Mount Kilimanjaro.

Here, not far from the Olduvai Gorge where some of the earliest evidence of humanity was found in the late 1950s, Tyson, America's second-largest food company and an icon of global industrial food production, was setting up a new site together with Irvine's, Africa's oldest industrial chicken producer. Their plan was nothing less than to fast-track the evolution of poultry in Africa by growing millions of genetically identical birds somewhere far away from people, pathogens and the possibility of disease.

Tysons and Irvine's are corporate giants with huge research and development budgets. Tysons alone rears, processes and sells over 11 billion chickens a year, mostly in the US to chains like McDonald's. If all went well, this remote farm on the African plain could expect soon to be sending 500,000 fertilised eggs a week to a sister hatchery on the Tanzanian coast, where many millions of one-day-old chicks would be sold to local farmers. In a few years' time, the Tanzanian operation would be rearing and exporting 1 million identical Cobb 500s a week to neighbouring Kenya, Rwanda, the Democratic Republic of Congo and other African countries. Motivated by both profit and a desire to improve life, the plan was to flood central Africa with these patented chickens, persuading tens of millions of people to forego the strong taste of native birds and turn to the milder, blander taste of the far cheaper Cobb 500.

When I was finally given permission to visit the farm in early 2019, it looked as if aliens had landed. The snows of Mount Kilimanjaro glistened above the clouds in the far distance and dozens of identical, low, 120-metre-long, twelve-metre-wide, shiny white steel and plastic sheds bristling with radio masts, tanks and communication towers had been incongruously and anonymously sited behind three-metre-high wire fences. As befits an American-owned enterprise setting up in Africa with chickens bred in the Netherlands to be sold on the international market for their meat, the works had been built by foreign labour.

The modern chicken is an industrial phenomenon. A parent hen will lay on average 192 eggs in its short fifteen-month life, more than twice as many as any backyard bird; a young broiler can grow from a day-old chick to a two-kilogram bird ready for the pot in just thirty-three days. The Cobb is now identically bred in 120 countries and is the first choice of most of the world's big poultry farmers and fast-food chains from McDonald's to Wendy's, KFC and Zaxby's.

Chicken is likely soon to overtake pork and beef to become the world's most popular meat, an essential part of the diet of billions of people. The UN's Food and Agriculture Organization estimated in 2002 that there were 19 billion chickens alive. Today there are probably 33 billion and our appetite for them is insatiable.[1]

The factory on the windswept plain was being run by Enzo, a young Brazilian vet who was deeply aware of the risks of keeping large numbers of birds in cramped conditions. Ever since intensive poultry farming started in earnest nearly 100 years ago, birds reared intensively have been found to be lame, weak, sick and injured, often suffering serious heart, bone and muscle disorders. Genetically identical, similarly aged, poorly fed and with their immune systems depressed by drugs, factory farming makes them perfectly susceptible to picking up, passing on and amplifying diseases.

Like all poultry breeders Enzo was terrified that avian flu might start on his farm. The merest hint of just a few of his birds showing symptoms like breathing problems and diarrhoea could mean having to kill possibly hundreds of thousands in hours. His mission, he said, was to eliminate the chance of them catching and passing on any disease. That meant preventing birds from coming into any contact with any wild bird, insect, mammal, rodent or human. The nightmare scenario was that a highly pathogenic disease might devastate a flock or, worse, emerge and spread to others.

Only after stripping, showering twice, brushing my teeth, washing my hair and donning special clothes – hat, mask, gloves and shoes – was I allowed to enter. The windowless buildings were built to be bird-, rat- and insect-proof, the water is purified, the surfaces disinfected, the air filtered and the climate and lighting computer-controlled. To get in requires nearly as many permissions, precautions and safety measures as entry to a high-security laboratory handling Ebola or Covid-19 pathogens.

All I could see when the sealed doors into the shed were opened were 100,000 or more identical white birds stretching several hundred metres into the distance; the only sound was the rumble of clucking hens, interspersed with the crowing of many hundreds of cocks. The lights were dimmed to reduce stress, the air was dry and circulating and the temperature cool. Food was delivered to the birds on conveyor belts.

The birds looked content. Up close, I could see why these chickens were known as 'nature's Arnold Schwarzeneggers' – they were all jutting chests, rippling thighs and big feet, genetically programmed to grow fast and eat only small quantities of cheap soya and maize. It was only when I got down to floor level that the cocks attacked. Feet out, wings flapping and beaks thrusting, they came at me hard. All I could do was yell and run.

* * *

We think we know flu. We have grown up with the sore throats, streaming noses and fevers it brings. We know that there are different strains and that each year one or more will circle the globe. We may not realise that it is likely to kill 36,000 mainly old people each year in the UK alone,[2] but we do know there are vaccines that protect against it, so we accept it as a miserable, but next to inevitable, occasional illness which may force us to spend time in bed in the winter months.

What we know and occasionally experience is 'seasonal' flu, which is local, mostly mild and more or less predictable. Seasonal influenza viruses spread throughout the world in a year or two, infecting 10 to 25 per cent of the world's population and causing some 290,000 to 650,000 deaths worldwide. With a world population of about 8 billion, the fatality rate is between 0.0036 per cent and 0.0081 per cent. No wonder seasonal influenza does not seem particularly dangerous.[3]

Pandemic flu, however, is altogether different – twenty times as dangerous and caused by the emergence of a new influenza virus to which there is little or no existing immunity in the human population. These pandemic flus appear roughly every thirty-five years and can be some of the most severe public health disasters any country ever has to face. A new flu virus is not just likely to infect up to half the world in a very short time but can be nearly as dangerous as Ebola or HIV/Aids, easily able to kill one in three – or more – of the people it infects.

Flu viruses are extraordinary. They originate in wild birds and are ancient, capricious and unstable, spawning many strains, variants and subtypes that can evolve and replicate by mutation or by mixing genes. They fascinate virologists because they can emerge and circulate in mammals, birds and humans until they evolve or mutate to be able to infect people who are immune to existing strains. They can be both the mildest of human and animal diseases and also the most severe. Some barely ruffle the feathers of an infected bird, while others can lead to a flock of 100,000 factory birds falling down dead in a few hours. Very occasionally one may jump from a bird to a human, and even more rarely one can jump from one human to another.

Technically, flu viruses are divided into four large families, A, B, C and D, and then into a bewildering alphabet soup of subtypes and variants based on the properties of their hemagglutinin (H) and neuraminidase (N) proteins. Types B and C circulate continuously and produce the mild seasonal symptoms many people experience every winter; type D infects mostly cattle, and only type A can produce a human pandemic. But because the type A viruses mutate so often, flu is now effectively a perpetually emerging disease, and one of the most contagious pathogens known, circulating widely without symptoms both in wild birds and in commercial flocks of geese, ducks, poultry, ostrich, chickens and pigs.

There have been possibly only fifteen human flu pandemics in the last 500 years, but there will inevitably be more because we have developed an insatiable appetite for poultry meat, and the way we farm birds raises our chances of a virus jumping into humans. Spurred by industrial-scale poultry producers, a global trading system that treats chicken as a commodity and a highly efficient global transport system, chicken – and to a lesser extent duck and turkey – has become by far the most common protein source for humans and the most likely source of new pandemics.

From possibly 3 million tonnes of poultry meat being reared fifty years ago, we now eat nearly 100 million tonnes a year.[4] Chicken consumption has grown by 70 per cent since 1990 alone and keeps on growing. Of the roughly 30 billion farm animals that are alive at any one point, some 23 billion are now chickens. The problem is that no one has any idea when or where another flu type will emerge, but by turning to birds for our most important source of meat protein, we are creating the conditions for another to emerge sooner rather than later.

* * *

The last great pandemic of the nineteenth century, known as the Russian flu, was a severe viral infection first identified in 1889 in Bukhara, the ancient, fabled city of myth and mosques on the Silk Road in what is now Uzbekistan. It was to be the world's first modern pandemic, notable for the speed at which it circled the world by public transport, and for its high visibility. It was the first to be followed closely by a newly emerging media. Newspapers of the time described it as a 'flu' and recorded how it spread rapidly westwards on the Trans-Caspian railway, which had only arrived in Bukhara the previous year. Carried by rail, it quickly reached Moscow and then London, where it killed Prince Albert Victor, the second in line to the British throne.

Crossing the Atlantic by steamship, it circled the world in a year, killing as many as 1 million people in a global population one sixth the size it is now. Without vaccines and with no treatments, the disease burned through communities, returning in wave after wave of infection for several more years until it became more or less endemic and disappeared.

But was it even the flu? There was little understanding of its origins at the time. Viruses had yet to be identified by science, and medical thinking was still fixated on miasma theory, which suggested that the weather created toxic air that poisoned people. Doubt about its viral origins was sown in 2005 when Belgian researchers led by the virologist Leen Vijgen compared the mutation rates of a human coronavirus known today as OC43 with another that infects cows. The two viruses were genetically close and appeared to have a common ancestor dating to about 1890. Possibly, they proposed, it was not a flu at all, but a coronavirus which emerged and then spread in cattle.[5]

There were plenty of cattle plagues around in the years leading up to the Russian flu pandemic, but there are other possibilities, says virologist Harald Bruessow, a researcher at KU Leuven in Belgium. He and his wife, also a microbiologist, ploughed through European historical records and found apparent references to it in cats, dogs and other animals but none in cattle. One report implicated a parrot, but otherwise, he says, they did not find any links to infections in birds.

But Bruessow's research suggests that the disease may not have originated in Bukhara at all, but in China, where ducks and geese had for centuries been kept by smallholder farmers in close contact with humans and from where vast flocks of migratory wild birds cross the world on what is known as the great Asian flyway – a series of migratory bird routes.[6]

'Cattle and horses might have served as intermediate hosts in 1889 but the arguments I saw in the historical records did not convince me of a bovine or equine origin for transmission of the 1889 pandemic. The epidemic was certainly favoured by the development of large cities with good railway and steamboat connections,' he said in an email exchange.

We may never know the 1889 pandemic's origins but thirty years later the single most fatal event in human history emerged from the chaos of the world's greatest war. Well-known war diseases like diarrhoea, measles, TB, dysentery, pneumonia and typhus all flourished from the start of hostilities in 1914, and the flooded, muddy trenches offered new maladies like trench foot, but by early 1918 an exceptionally severe flu virus had emerged to strike up to one in four of the millions of soldiers on the 800-kilometre long Western Front.

Short of genetic material, researchers have three theories about how the 1918 flu epidemic started. For some it is a toss-up between British army camps in Aldershot,[7] and a chicken farm in Kansas that passed it to one of the US's army's vast transit camps where soldiers gathered before going to Europe.[8] A third group thinks that it may have sailed to Europe with the 96,000 Chinese labourers who were brought in to work behind the British and French lines in 1917, even as an unidentified fever was raging in China.

However it arrived, when presented with millions of overcrowded animals and humans living hugger-mugger in unsanitary conditions on the front lines, the virus – now identified as H1N1 – spread, mutated and flourished. Vast quantities of food were required to feed the soldiers and all the many transit, training and frontline army camps, each housing 25–35,000 people, were ordered to set up their own pig and livestock farms. But with exhausted, often gassed and wounded men eating poorly cooked food and living with stressed, domesticated animals, it is more than possible that the flu emerged, mutated and spread uncontained in the camps, says biologist and historian David Payne.[9]

'[The flu's] genesis probably lay in the mutation of avian type influenza from Asia which jumped the species via pigs to arrive in the crowded military base camps of the USA and Europe. There was an extraordinarily high mortality rate of twenty times the norm for influenza. Death often occurred within a few hours. In many of the cases that did survive the critical first few days of the influenza attack, death was precipitated by a rampant secondary infection by pneumonia bacteria,' wrote Payne for the Western Front Association.[10]

Wherever it started, the first wave of infection killed hundreds of thousands of young soldiers, but the second wave, carried to all points on earth by the world's armies returning to their countries when the war ended, was cataclysmic, ripping through defenceless communities from Alaska to Australia and Scotland to South Africa.[11] One in three people in the US may have been infected and possibly 20–50 million died worldwide – far more than the 16 million thought to have died in the combat itself, and probably many more than from the successive bubonic plagues of the Middle Ages.

* * *

The consensus now is that the 1918 pandemic was created by the stress of war combined with the overcrowding of humans and diseased animals.[12] Strangely it seemed to affect rural communities much more than urban ones, possibly because people living in cities had acquired some immunity from earlier H1-like outbreaks, perhaps including the 1889 pandemic.[13]

The combination of war and flu led to a cascade of social and cultural changes that are still with us. The move to cities increased, the number of land workers reduced, farms became larger and a more mechanised and global industrial food system began to replace traditional farming societies. As cities grew, so diets changed, the production of meat intensified and the nature of disease also altered. The virus never entirely disappeared; instead it spawned hundreds more smaller, shorter-lived epidemics over the following years.

It took nearly forty years for the next flu pandemic to emerge. By 1957 the global population had almost doubled to 2.8 billion people and the flu that emerged in duck flocks in Guizhou, southern China, is believed to have killed 1–4 million people. The first cases of what became known as Asian flu were reported in late 1956 and early in 1957 in Singapore. Virologists raced to understand whether it was a new strain or simply a descendant of the previous 1918–19 pandemic influenza virus. It was the former.

Within weeks it was rampant in China and Hong Kong, where it reportedly infected 250,000 people, 10 per cent of the population. By June it had spread to India, the UK and USA and within five months of its outbreak in Hong Kong it had circled the globe. 'As an entirely new strain there was no immunity in the populace and the first vaccines were not distributed until August in the US and October in the UK, and then on an extremely limited basis,' wrote the health journalist Claire Jackson.[14]

Later research found that the virus was a 're-assortment', or mixing, of avian and human influenza viruses. Archive BBC recordings suggest that it infected possibly 10 million people and left whole continents wheezing and sneezing, if not heading for hospitals.[15] In 2020 Wellcome Trust medical historian Mark Honigsbaum wrote in the *Lancet* how there were no conspiracy theories, or need for social distancing, 'For most people it was private. For the very great majority, it wasn't that significant. In 1957 there was … no possibility of intervention. There was not a lot that people could do to protect themselves or treat it.'[16]

From then on, flu pandemics came faster. It took just eleven more years for the fourth modern flu pandemic to arrive and circle the earth. Again, the 1968 pandemic almost certainly started in a mainland Chinese poultry farm, but this time it was named after Hong Kong, where it arrived in July. This virus was a direct descendant of the 1957 Asian flu and was both highly transmissible and severe, infecting nearly 500,000 people in its first two weeks, reaching the US in December and Europe shortly afterwards. Once again, war played a role in spreading it around the world. The virus entered California via troops returning from the Vietnam War.

But 1968–69 was a tumultuous social and political time and the international media paid little attention. The war, the Paris riots, which were shaking governments in Western Europe, and the space race all consumed the media. In this time of great cultural upheaval, possibly 10 million people or more were infected, and between 1 and 4 million died. Apollo 8 commander Frank Borman went down with it during his mission in December 1968 but the stock market did not crash, schools did not close, there was no lockdown and people carried on working.

* * *

Enzo's attention to biosafety on his chicken farm on that windswept African plain in 2019 can be traced back to events in Hong Kong twenty years later when the fourth great global flu epidemic almost happened. Even as China was preparing to take back from the British the densely packed city-state of 7 million people in January 1997, an outbreak of bird flu struck three small chicken farms in the rural New Territories district of the colony.

That it did not turn into a catastrophic pandemic of the same severity as the 1918 flu is entirely thanks to the heroic actions of a small group of vets and doctors who recognised the risks, knew what to do and persuaded the authorities, who were entirely new in Hong Kong, to act decisively. The strain that emerged was particularly nasty. In just a few days more than 5,000 birds turned zombie-like and started laying eggs without shells and collapsing with blood clots. It was traumatic and economically catastrophic for farmers and market traders, who had never seen anything like it.

Because bird flu can flare up unexpectedly among chickens, ducks and turkeys in different ways at different times, this outbreak was again mostly missed by the press and governments. To be fair, there had been more than a dozen similar outbreaks of bird flu around the world in the previous twenty years, but no humans seemed to be infected and the natural barrier between birds and humans which prevents the spillover of disease between different species did not seem to be threatened.

But in early May 1997, Lam Hoi-ka, a three-year-old boy with no history of illness, was rushed by his parents to Queen Elizabeth Hospital in Kowloon in the New Territories district with a sore throat, fever and severe stomach pain. It was immediately diagnosed as influenza but doctors were baffled when, shortly after being admitted, he developed pneumonia. Then his lungs, liver and kidneys began to fail. Inside a week he had inexplicably died.[17]

It fell to Professor Kennedy Shortridge, a lanky young Australian microbiologist at the University of Hong Kong, to isolate the virus that had attacked young Lam Hoi-ka.[18] Tests showed it had indeed been a highly pathogenic Influenza A virus, but not one of the sixteen known subtypes or variants. Specimens were immediately sent to virologists in London, the US Centers for Disease Control in Atlanta and the Netherlands, and by August it was confirmed that H5N1, as it had been named, had not only jumped directly from birds to humans but looked as if it had passed between humans.

Virologists were shocked, immediately grasping the significance of a new strain of flu crossing from a bird to kill a human and then passing between humans. This was one of the first times that an avian Influenza A virus of any subtype causing respiratory infection and human death had been documented. Ominously, an important source of food was now the source of a zoonotic infectious disease that stood to become a potential global health threat.

Mike Davis, a respected American journalist writing in 2003, reported near panic among virologists investigating the samples at the CDC in Atlanta. 'Horrified scientists, who had never seen such a rapid killer, immediately donned biohazard containment suits and dosed themselves with antivirals. A majority of the research community now decided that H5N1 research should be analysed in one of the world's highest safety "Level 4" laboratories. A single mutation – a difference of just three amino acids – had apparently allowed the bird virus to open the lock on human cells and infect the child.'[19] He reported how one anonymous US scientist had said: 'It reproduced much faster than ordinary flu strains, and in cells that ordinary flu strains couldn't live in, and if you grew it in eggs, it killed them.'

Virologist Nancy Cox, who went on to direct the CDC's Influenza Division in Atlanta, was equally shocked: 'We had the dogma that there was an extremely high barrier between the host and the species that prevented avian flu viruses from infecting humans and vice versa. We had to get rid of those ideas, one by one, this situation was new,' she told Davis.

Until then, it had been mostly understood that all the many subtypes of Influenza A virus were incompatible with human receptors and that it needed an intermediary host, possibly a pig, to enable the virus to move to humans. This one was clearly different. 'It was supposed to only cause disease in birds. This is like the clock striking thirteen,' Stephen Morse, director of the Center for Public Health Preparedness at Columbia University, told *Newsweek* in 2004.[20]

Back in Hong Kong, the trail had gone cold. Lam Hoi-ka had reportedly played with a few baby chickens at his school and possibly one of them had passed it to him, but they were long dead now. There had been no more cases or outbreaks, and no reports from mainland China. By August 1997 the virus had seemingly disappeared. Shortridge and colleagues held their breath and dared to hope the case was an exception, a fluke, possibly a warning. The world, it seemed, might for the first time have averted a pandemic, if not prevented one.

But Hong Kong did not have long to wait. In November 1997, a full five months after Lam Hoi-ka had died, Shortridge's fear that a human pandemic was on the point of breaking out was confirmed when Hong Kong farmers found chickens losing their appetite, coughing, sneezing and acting strangely.

Even more seriously, within days, a 37-year-old man from Kowloon who had had no known contact with chickens or the young lad also fell ill, followed three days later by a girl from the new town of Ma On Shan. Over the next six weeks eighteen people were infected by the H5N1 virus, of whom six died. The source of infection appeared to be live-poultry markets where chickens, ducks, geese, quail and other birds were sold.

Shortridge and colleagues understood what was at stake. The virus was nearly as dangerous as HIV/Aids, Ebola or Marburg, liable to kill 30–50 per cent of all the people it infected, and therefore far more dangerous than H1N1, the flu that had killed more than 50 million people in the Spanish flu pandemic of 1918. Moreover, tests of chickens for sale in the Hong Kong poultry markets showed that one in five birds were infected with H5N1 viruses. H5N1 seemed to be an order of magnitude more lethal than every other known human influenza virus on record.

The Chinese authorities, who had taken over the administration of Hong Kong from the British only months earlier, were initially overwhelmed by the implications. To their credit, they were persuaded by Shortridge and other scientists to act fast and decisively with no concern for the city's immediate economy. Instead, they ordered the immediate slaughter of all 1.5 million chickens and several hundred thousand other domestic fowl in the colony. 'We don't know what will happen with this virus. We've had no contact with it before. For all we know it might go to humans and completely fade away,' said Shortridge.[21]

So it was that on 28 December 1997, nearly 4,000 people fanned out across the territory to collect and kill by hand all the former colony's chickens, ducks, geese, quails and pigeons in the 160 poultry farms and 1,000 market stalls, shops and wholesalers.[22] The bodies of the birds were disinfected, wrapped in plastic and taken to landfills. There were no further outbreaks and it seemed that a pandemic had been stamped out. It was said to be mutating so fast that it was very close to being able to transmit from human to human.

Hong Kong widely suspected China to be the source of the virus but China has never officially acknowledged that it had an H5N1 problem. However, documents prior to the 1997 outbreak revealed that its Ministry of Health had requested H5N1 re-agents from the World Health Organization, which are used to test for the presence of antibodies to the virus. This suggests, although it was never confirmed, that China at least suspected this type of influenza might be afflicting its poultry, but did not yet have the means to test for it.

What had happened, it emerged years later, was that in the early spring of 1996 several outbreaks of a deadly disease had struck a goose farm near Foshan, a small rural town about eighty kilometres west of the fast-growing city of Guangzhou, 190 kilometres from Hong Kong. Two viruses, called A/goose/Guangdong/1/1996 and A/goose/Guangdong/2/1996, were isolated at the Chinese National Influenza Centre and the disease was officially named H5N1 in 1997. Shortridge's suspicions that it had originated on a poultry farm has been proved correct. Whether H5N1 had spread to the domesticated geese from a passing wild bird or vice versa will never be known, but the H5 virus went on to become one of the worst pandemics ever seen in wildlife, over the next twenty-five years forcing the culling of billions of poultry and the agonising death of untold numbers of wild birds and other species.

* * *

H5N1 had not been stamped out. It lay low for nearly three years but in 2001 and again in 2002 it was found in mild form in wild birds and ducks in southern China. The next year it returned to Hong Kong markets, almost certainly via the thousands of live birds imported daily from the mainland. The same year new subtypes were found and the disease caused huge outbreaks in several large poultry farms in China, South Korea and Vietnam.

Clearly H5N1 was on the march, but in 2004 the worst happened. The disease exploded across Southeast Asia and started killing people again. More than 100 million chickens and poultry in thousands of villages and farms throughout the region had to be slaughtered, and in the US a young member of the Senate Committee on Foreign Relations warned of 'alarming developments'. Barack Obama wrote in the *New York Times*: 'The virus has been detected in mammals that have never been previously infected including tigers, leopards and domestic cats. This spread suggests that the virus is mutating and could eventually emerge in a form that is readily transmitted between humans, leading to a full-blown pandemic.'[23]

Obama had been well briefed. Over the next five years the fast-mutating highly pathogenic H5N1 spread round the world with major outbreaks in more than seventy countries, mainly in wild birds. It was also found in ferrets, mice and badgers.

Sporadically it kept appearing in humans. By November 2020, there had been 861 cases and 465 human deaths, suggesting a mortality rate of more than 50 per cent, similar to Ebola. So far it has been largely confined to people working with poultry.

'No one knows whether it will evolve into a pandemic strain but flu viruses constantly change,' said Japanese virologist Yoshiro Kawaoka, who has worked on the virus almost since it emerged.[24]

Even more concerning is that H5N1 is just one strain of highly pathogenic avian flu now circling an increasingly infected globe. In the past twenty years at least twelve novel flu viruses have mutated and jumped the host-species barrier in both wild birds and poultry farms. From just a few subtypes identified one hundred years ago there are now H6N1, H7N9, H5N6, H5N8, H7N7, H5N9, H5N2, H7N1, H9N2 and others. They have emerged not only in China but across Europe, Australia, the US and North America.

As I write this in the summer of 2022, the H5 strain has exploded and its variants have been found in more than a hundred countries, with at least five, including H5N1, H5N2, H5N8 and H7N9, circulating strongly. One, known as H7N9, came the closest to becoming a new pandemic, killing at least three people when it emerged close to Lake Poyang in China in 2013.

Within a year it was mutating frequently, spreading to chicken and duck farms in fourteen Chinese provinces and to Taiwan, Malaysia and Canada. By 2020 there had been more than 1,500 cases, mainly in mainland China, and more than 500 deaths, suggesting that one in three people infected with it die.[25]

H5N8 is now the variant of most concern because it can infect other birds so easily. It emerged first on a duck farm in South Korea and soon spread to other poultry farms. It has now exploded, with hundreds of outbreaks in commercial farms across Europe and Asia and among wild bird flocks. Close on 100 million poultry in seventeen countries have died or had to be culled. Each outbreak increases the chances of a strain acquiring human-to-human transmission capability, making the emergence of a full-blown human pandemic more likely. For some experts it is a matter of when, not if.

INTENSIVE CARE

Why do pandemics so often start in southern China? That was the question Australian microbiologist Kennedy Shortridge kept asking as he worked in the laboratories of the Hong Kong University Hospital in the 1980s. Why had the Asian flu in 1957 and the 1968 Hong Kong flu pandemics, as well as SARS and so many other emerging diseases in both humans and wildlife, all seemed to originate there? Was it the climate, the history, the culture, the health system or the way people farmed animals? Could it be linked to environmental change or politics? 'Influenza research is a continuing detective story, with all the intrigue of an Agatha Christie novel,' he wrote in 1999.[1]

Haunted by his mother's stories of the catastrophic 1918 flu pandemic when horse-drawn carts piled with dead bodies passed through Mount Isa, his small home town in Queensland, Australia, Shortridge had arrived in Hong Kong in 1972 after studying flu viruses in London. It was the right place and time for a flu researcher. Not only had the 1957 Asian H2N2 and the 1968 Hong Kong H3N2 pandemics both started in or close to the city-state, but the laboratories he was to work in had led global research into their emergence. His papers and reports show how he threw himself into the work, collecting and monitoring viruses from chicken, geese and ducks found in markets and farms throughout the colony.

Lab work fascinated Shortridge but it was when he started travelling beyond the bubble of Hong Kong island to Guangdong and other mainland Chinese states and conferring with Chinese scientists that he really began to understand how human activities determined where and when zoonotic diseases could emerge and spread.

Back in the 1970s southern China was crowded but desperately poor, its overwhelmingly rural population living much as it had done for centuries. Families were mostly small-scale rice farmers, habitually letting their few ducks and pigs range freely. In this deeply conservative, barely changing environment where people and domestic poultry and pigs lived cheek by jowl, much as they had done several thousand years before, Shortridge found it unsurprising that people would have built immunity to bird viruses. The great Poyang lake and other wetlands north of Hong Kong were prime stopovers for the huge flocks of migrating geese, storks, ducks, swans, herons and egrets on what ornithologists call the great 'East Asian Flyway' between Siberia and Australia. Many of the wild birds overwinter every year and mix freely with free-range domestic birds.

Southern China and its innumerable ponds and rice paddy fields, pigs and poultry, he hypothesised, was a 'viral soup', an evolutionary hotspot of human and avian influenza. Because pigs could be infected by both poultry flu and human flu, genetic material from each of the three species could combine and form new flu strains. Moreover, the molecular and genetic evidence suggested that chickens were not the natural host for influenza so much as the domestic duck, raised in great numbers in southern China since antiquity.

But if people had been living close to ducks for millennia without undue problems, something had to have changed for so many new diseases to emerge from China in such a short time, he reasoned. The answer, he became convinced, was both under his nose and global. Poultry farming in southern China was ceasing to be a small-scale peasant activity, and had been intensifying worldwide since the Great War. Enormous political change was also seeing China open to the world, even as its human population was exploding. The combination of the historic 'viral soup' with the modern loss of nature, the expansion and industrialisation of farming and the move to cities made it inevitable that viruses would spill over from animals to humans more frequently and make pandemics like bird flu and SARS more likely.

Shortridge's thirty-year work in Hong Kong coincided with China's headlong dash to industrial domination. Southern China in particular was changing fast, with millions of people leaving the land to live and work in cities like Guangzhou. As China's version of capitalism unfolded, the physical world of the most populous country on earth was changing dramatically. Forests were being felled, wetlands converted into farmland, wild lands fragmented – and since there was more money around and better transportation, people were turning to once-scarce meat.

When he arrived in 1972 the average Chinese ate less than five kilograms of meat a year. By the time he left in 2002, it was more than thirty kilograms. In 1968 about 13 million chickens were being reared at any one time in China. By 1997, when he and his colleagues had persuaded the new Chinese government in Hong Kong to cull millions of poultry to avoid H5N1 avian flu, it was close to 1 billion.[2]

People had not lost a taste for freshly killed meat but the small backyard peasant farmer with a few birds for his pot and a few to sell at the local wildlife or wet market was being left behind, unable to compete with the giant poultry-rearing sheds, abattoirs and processing plants setting up on the edges of China's burgeoning cities.

Shortridge realised that these social and ecological changes were making southern China ground zero for a future pandemic to emerge. In the 1980s he had established that avian influenza and human influenza viruses had reasserted themselves in pigs, helping to explain the swine flu virus of 1957, which had mysteriously disappeared from humans but carried on in pigs.

Now he and his colleagues started to warn that the closeness of human habitations to the farms in southern China made it a perfect place for a bird flu virus to cross the species barrier to man.[3] 'Quite simply the region has a permanent gene pool of avian influenza viruses year-round. This is as a consequence of the domestication of the duck as a source of these viruses around 4,500 years ago in the fertile southeastern region of the country and subsequent intensification and spread of duck raising as an adjunct to rice farming around the start of the Ching Dynasty in 1644. By contrast, an avian influenza gene pool similar to the one in southern China does not exist anywhere else in the world,' he concluded.[4]

So when, in April 2009, a new strain of H1N1 influenza virus killed two children in San Diego, California, and was traced to an intensive pig farm over the border in Mexico, the finger of blame naturally pointed east to China – home of half the world's pigs and where influenza viruses were known to jump among birds, human and pigs. Dubbed swine flu, it was the first pandemic of the twenty-first century and governments rushed to find vaccines. But as it rapidly spread around the world, eventually killing up to 575,000 people,[5] epidemiologists struggled to explain how a virus in an Asian pig could spark a pandemic that began in humans in Mexico. 'We admitted it did not make sense,' said Martha Nelson, a biologist at the US National Institute of Allergy and Infectious Diseases.

She and a handful of other pathogen hunters met in 2010 in Belgium. 'We sketched out on a whiteboard the possible scenarios for the pandemic's origins, each of which seemed far-fetched. Could "patient zero" be a Chinese hog farmer who flew to Mexico? … Or did an Asian pig make its way to Mexico some time before the pandemic? … No one knew.'

It took years of genetic sampling and digging into the records of global pig movements for Nelson and her colleagues to show how the world's multi-billion dollar pig trade was spreading influenza. What had happened was that, following the 1994 North American Free Trade Agreement (NAFTA) which liberalised US and Mexico trade, millions of pigs, some of which carried H1N1, had been trucked into Mexico, where labour was cheaper. At the same time, Mexico-based factory farms had independently imported European pigs with other swine flu viruses. The American- and European-origin viruses had exchanged genetic material to create the brand-new pathogen that jumped to humans in 2009. Moreover, humans had helped spread the disease not just among themselves but back to pigs, ensuring it continued to circulate.

Nelson was shocked. 'The global pandemic that scientists had long feared had finally arrived, only no one predicted it would come from North America. For most of the 20th century, influenza was not a problem for pig farmers. But as agricultural production of pigs expanded and modernized at a blistering pace, with backyard farms being displaced by large commercial operations all over the world, the opportunity for viral intermixing grew exponentially and cases of flu in swine began to climb,' she wrote in 2022.[6]

China may have been the historical hotbed of avian and pig flu, as Shortridge had proposed, but no longer.

* * *

Kennedy Shortridge died in 2020, just as Covid-19 was starting to circle the world and HPAI avian influenza was starting to decimate wild bird populations on three continents. His linking of avian flu pandemics to the profound industrial, social and ecological changes taking place in China helped the world understand both how and why infectious diseases emerge and spread.

His death also coincided with the outbreak of a highly pathogenic flu in a giant poultry farm near the city of Astrakhan in southern Russia.[7] Workers at the Vladimirskaya plant were shocked when more than 100,000 chickens housed in large sheds started to collapse and die. Tests conducted hurriedly by the state research centre showed that a relatively new strain of lethal avian flu known as H5N8 was circulating, and within days 900,000 more birds at the Vladimirskaya plant were slaughtered to prevent a wider epidemic.[8]

But the Astrakhan incident was not like the many thousands of other outbreaks of H5N8 that had devastated commercial chicken, duck and turkey flocks across nearly fifty countries over the previous few years.[9] When 150 workers at the Astrakhan farm were tested, five women and two men were found to have caught the disease, albeit mildly. It was the first time that H5N8 had ever been known to jump from birds to humans.

The WHO was alerted, but with the Covid-19 pandemic crowding out international news, little attention was paid even when Anna Popova, the chief consumer adviser to the Russian Federation, went on TV to warn 'with a degree of probability' that human-to-human transmission of H5N8 would evolve soon and that work should start immediately on making a vaccine. 'Only time will tell how soon future mutations will allow it to overcome this barrier. The discovery of this strain gives the world time to prepare for possible mutations,' she said.[10]

Popova was right to warn the world about a new human pandemic starting on a poultry farm. More than a dozen new flu virus subtypes and variants now regularly rattle around the world's big chicken and duck plants, any one of which could evolve to become the next H5N1 or human flu. H1N1 gave the world the Spanish flu in 1918, and H3N2 avian flu in 2003, but now H1N2v, H3N2v, H3N8, H5N1, H6N1, H7N1, H7N3, H7N7, H7N9 and H9 have all been identified. Ominously, human cases are picking up, too. Since October 2020, there have been more than 3,000 outbreaks of avian flu on four continents, with hundreds of millions of birds having to be slaughtered. The risk to humans is still very low, but sixty-four cases of four novel strains have been recorded in China, Laos, Russia, Nigeria and the UK. All have been in people in close contact with poultry.

The virus subvariants are mostly 'low pathogenic', and not dangerous at all to domesticated birds, but if given the chance can mutate and 're-assort' themselves with other viruses introduced by other birds or humans. The risk is that one may eventually mutate into a virus that is transmissible to – or, worse, between – humans. Two subtypes in particular, H5 and H7, have been found to be mutating the fastest. Both sporadically cross into humans, causing deaths mostly among people working close to them, as in Astrakhan.

While governments and industry routinely blame wild birds for transmitting avian flu viruses to domesticated flocks,[11] evidence has mounted that intensive farms are now the melting pots for new, potentially deadly viruses.[12] UN bodies, academics[13] and epidemiologists all recognise that there are now unprecedented numbers of diseases like salmonella, avian and swine flu, bovine TB, African swine fever, brucellosis and SARS emerging in humans and animals, with around 75 per cent of them linked to farming or the eating of poultry, cattle, pigs or wild animals.[14]

Some of this disease emergence is simply because keeping genetically similar animals in stressful conditions allows disease to rip through a flock or herd of animals easily. Poor welfare weakens resistance and overcrowding increases the chances of a disease spreading. But large, intensive farms with tens of thousands of genetically identical animals can also act as an 'epidemiological bridge' between wildlife and human infections.[15]

I called Dutch virologist Marion Koopmans, a leading avian flu researcher and one of the WHO's nine-person team chosen to investigate the emergence of Covid-19 in Wuhan. 'How far does intensive poultry farming now threaten to make avian flu a global pandemic?' I asked.

'Having some birds infected here and there in the wild is a different level of human health risk than having the same infection burn through a high-density poultry farm with thousands of birds. But over the past few years we have seen a massive shift in the ecology of H5 avian influenza which is now present in wild birds across Europe, and spreading into the Americas. So here, the pressure comes from wildlife, and the level of biosecurity of farms is a critical factor', she told me.

So was H5 now out of control and liable to affect both wild and domesticated bird populations on a global scale? 'I am afraid that is a likely scenario,' she said.

According to the UN's Food and Agricultural Organization,[16] the danger in farms with densely packed animals is that 'a pathogen may turn into a hyper-virulent disease agent; in monocultures involving mass rearing of genetically identical animals … an emerging hyper-virulent pathogen will rapidly spread within a flock or herd.'[17]

American biologist Rob Wallace from a group of researchers called the Agroecology and Rural Economics Research Corps has advised the UN and governments, but his persistent warnings for years about the danger of factory farms were routinely dismissed as 'unscientific' and 'misleading the public' by the authorities and industry. However, new research and the arrival of Covid-19 have changed the debate.

Wallace comes from a family of virologists and is steeped in the political ecology of disease and how and why it emerges. Like Kennedy Shortridge twenty-five years earlier, he focuses on the social context in which farming is practised. The liberalisation of trade and dismantling of tariffs, subsidies for industrial farming and the methods used have fed millions of people, but are together driving disease, he says.[18]

The modern poultry industry, consolidated into a handful of giant corporations, risks disaster, he argues. In just fifty years, the pursuit of efficiency and profit, he suggests, has developed vast flocks of genetically identical chickens and ducks. By avoiding natural selection or any accidental breeding with wild birds, and breeding for qualities like size of breast or speed of growth,[19] they are dicing not just with the death of birds, but of humans and other animals. 'Broilers and layers alike are unable to reproduce on site and evolve. In other words, the failure to accumulate natural resistance to circulating pathogens is built into the industrial model before a single outbreak of disease occurs,' he says.[20]

Starting around 2016, he writes in an email, 'multiple outbreaks of deadly H5 bird flu started decimating poultry across Europe, Asia, and the Middle East. Avian and swine influenza strains have ramped up the rate of their evolution, spillover, and deadliness to animals and humans alike. Influenza's infiltration into industrial livestock and poultry is now so complete that these farms are their own source [of disease]. The virus is able to infect a broader range of host species, now including the poultry that global agribusiness raises in the billions.'[21]

With more than 20 billion chickens[22] and nearly 700 million pigs alive at any one time, the chance of new flu strains and variants emerging in factory farms and spilling over to humans is high.[23] 'When given nearly infinite opportunities to evolve and spill over into humans the evolution of the rare deadly influenza that can easily transmit human-to-human bends toward inevitable,' says Wallace.

The scale of industrial farming is now determining disease outbreaks, he believes. 'The more food for flu available, the deadlier the strains that win out. It used to be that we were hit just by the H1s, 2s and 3s [variants]. Now we're up into the H5s, 6s, 7s, and 9s. That doesn't bode well for pandemic planning, as we have little to no standing herd immunity to these new re-assortments.'[24]

Wallace concludes that industrial farms are becoming disease factories. He draws on research by epidemiologist and avian flu researcher Marius Gilbert and others at the Université Libre de Bruxelles in Belgium which shows how farms with tens of thousands of birds can now act as their own reservoirs of disease by helping to 'convert' mild flu strains into highly pathogenic ones. In one study of thirty-nine documented cases where the H5 and H7 strains converted to high deadliness, all but a very few occurred on large-scale poultry farms.[25]

Gilbert, Wallace and other epidemiologists have developed Shortridge's arguments, proposing that humans shape their own disease ecology and that the root problems of health are now social as much as they are viral. Rather than blame China for the emergence of flus, it makes more sense to look at the industrial model which generates the disease, suggests Wallace.

'Was the West Africa Ebola epidemic caused by Ebola virus or by the dismantling of public health infrastructure in the countries where it emerged, following years of structural adjustment? What's the agent? What's the cause?' asks Gilbert, and answers: 'The popular narrative of deadly viruses emerging from wildlife reservoirs distracts attention from the more important social, economic and cultural forces that … lead to epidemics.' It is the rapid intensification of poultry farming[26] which is now actually making bird flu viruses more dangerous.[27] 'There is clearly a link,' he says, 'between the emergence of highly pathogenic avian influenza viruses and intensified poultry production systems.'

Research into the human pathogens carried in farmed animals and the threats they pose is fast expanding. Oxford University professor of microbial genomics and evolution Samuel K. Sheppard has shown how keeping animals penned together for most of their lives triggers genetic changes in common bugs like campylobacter, which are now widespread in poultry and pigs and cattle. Intensive farming practices provide the perfect environment for bacteria[28] and viruses,[29] 'to merge, mutate, and then jump into humans', increasing the risk of epidemics, he told me in 2021.[30]

'There are an estimated 1.5 billion cattle on Earth, each producing around 30 kg of manure each day; if just 20 percent of these are carrying Campylobacter, that amounts to a huge potential public health risk. Over the past few decades, there have been several viruses and pathogenic bacteria that have switched species from wild animals to humans: HIV started in monkeys; H5N1 came from birds; now Covid-19 is suspected to have come from bats. Our work shows that environmental change and increased contact with farm animals has caused bacterial infections to cross over to humans, too.'[31]

The stakes have become higher as the full cost of a modern pandemic like Covid-19 are seen, says medical doctor and historian Michael Greger, author of the book *Bird Flu: A Virus of Our Own Hatching*.[32] Greger argues that there have been three eras of human disease: the first, when we started to domesticate animals about 10,000 years ago and were infected with their diseases, like measles and chickenpox; then in the eighteenth and nineteenth centuries, the industrial revolution led to epidemics of diabetes, obesity, heart disease and cancer; and now, agricultural intensification is leading to zoonotic, or animal-borne, diseases such as bird flu, salmonella, MERS, Nipah and Covid-19.

In evolutionary terms, rearing poultry, cattle and pigs in high-intensity, crowded, confined, entirely unnatural conditions may be the most profound alteration of the human–animal relationship in 10,000 years. 'We are seeing an unprecedented explosion in outbreaks of new viruses, which have the potential to be much worse than Covid. The next pandemic may be more of an unnatural disaster of our own making. A pandemic of even moderate impact may result in the single biggest human disaster ever [and] has the potential to redirect world history,' Greger says.[33]

I called Professor Sheppard again in October 2022 after finding gannets, shags and other sea birds washed up dead on beaches in the Isles of Scilly in the far southwest of Britain. The highly pathogenic H5N1 avian flu strain which had originated in the intensive goose farm in Guangdong province in 1996 and had later escaped into the wild bird populations of Asia was now raging out of control and decimating commercial flocks as well as wild bird colonies across Europe, North America and South Africa. The scale of this pandemic was unprecedented. Already it had infected over a hundred avian species, killing around a hundred million birds, but now it had been confirmed in foxes, skunks, bobcats, seals and opossums in North America and was showing no sign of stopping. It was potentially catastrophic for wildlife, but beyond advising people not to touch infected animals, governments and conservationists were helpless. Just as with Covid-19, a new virus had been let loose and no one had any idea what damage might result as it continued to mutate.

Sheppard linked the avian flu wildlife pandemic back to the way humans farmed, and was adamant that intensive animal rearing had to be scaled back or drastically changed if humans and wildlife were to thrive together. The explosion in the number of animals being bred to feed ever-expanding, wealthier human populations was changing the speed at which viruses and bacteria were evolving, he told me:

> Livestock, especially chickens, cattle and pigs, are now by far the most common animals on earth. Because of the sheer size of these host niches with many millions of individual animals, viruses and bacteria inevitably spill over into the environment and into wild animal species with potentially disastrous results. However, this is only part of the problem. The way evolution works is that as population sizes increase, so does the efficiency by which adapted strains emerge. Put another way, not only

does a large group of animals have more pathogens, but
they evolve faster. Any way you look at it, intensive livestock
production is inherently problematic.[34]

Alarm bells rang in late 2022 when hundreds of mink packed
closely together on a Spanish farm started dying. Veterinarians at
first thought it was Covid-19, known to infect mink, but it was
H5N1, or bird flu, which was rampaging among avian populations
across Europe and had possibly spread from a nearby colony. What
was worrisome was that mink are susceptible to both human and
bird flus, and the H5N1 virus had picked up several new mutations
on the intensive farm, at least one of which had enabled it to spread
more easily between mammals.[35]

Another hurdle preventing bird flu from spreading both to and
then between humans had seemingly been removed. The mink were
culled, the farm workers placed in quarantine and the outbreak
snuffed out. But virologists all over the world were left in no doubt
that bird flu could mutate and recombine into a human-infecting
virus, and that a new, long-feared global flu pandemic was closer
than ever.

Marion Koopmans, director of the Department of Virology
at the Erasmus Medical Centre in Rotterdam, whom I spoke
to earlier, warned that H5N1 was evolving and could jump to
humans. She told the BBC: 'This virus is now more or less global
in birds ... and we have reports of infections in foxes, seals and
other mammals. It doesn't mean that we are looking at the start of
a human epidemic, or even worse, a pandemic, but it is a warning
sign that these viruses are capable of infecting mammals, and large
groups of animals provide the opportunity for a virus to evolve,
and that's not something we should allow.'

CITY ILLS

At five in the wild, wet morning of 12 June 1956, the 1,100-tonne SS *Warri* coastal steamer, bound for London from Sapele with a cargo of palm oil pine kernels, misjudged a sandbar and foundered on the West African coast. It started breaking up in the heavy surf and listing heavily to port. Captain Alan Thomas ordered the crew to abandon ship.

They were fortunate that the *Warri* had run aground close to Iwerekun, a small village just thirty kilometres from Lagos, then the colonial capital of Nigeria. No lives were lost thanks to the kindness of the villagers but it was an arduous and dangerous three-day trek to Lagos by canoe and on foot through swamps, mangrove forests and lagoons to reach the city. 'The journey proved highly adventurous and not a little hazardous,' Thomas told the *Warri*'s owners.[1]

That stretch of wild coast is now part of Lagos city and some of Africa's most expensive real estate, lined with hotels, beach clubs, bars and apartment blocks. The village where the *Warri* had beached had long been swallowed by Lagos as the ramshackle city of 250,000 people in 1956 mushroomed into Africa's most populous city, with more than 25 million mostly young people today. Now it covers several thousand square kilometres, and is one end of an urban corridor stretching a thousand kilometres west to Abidjan in Côte d'Ivoire. Vibrant, fast, often frantic, it is a new world, albeit with two-thirds of its people living in overcrowded slums without access to clean water or sanitation.

Its well-connected rich and middle-class population of frequent travellers regularly imports and exports pathogens to and from the rest of the world, while its poor struggle to cope with them.

* * *

Urbanisation in Africa and Asia is unprecedented, matched only by the speed of growth of major cities in Europe and the US in the nineteenth century. As it did then, it is utterly changing the landscape of global health and disease, driving what people eat and how they move around and live. A further 3 billion people – the population of another China and India – are expected to be alive by 2100 and nearly all will live in what are now low- and middle-income African and Asian cities. It is here that epidemiologists expect diseases to catch hold and spread around the globe, because there is nothing pathogens like better than poverty and crowded, unhygienic places.

Disease has always shaped cities and determined their development. Athens and Rome dramatically declined in size after pandemics hollowed them out. The Aztec capital of Tenochtitlan reputedly collapsed under the burden of many Old World diseases brought by conquistadors. Cholera and typhoid made Europe's cities install sophisticated water and sanitation systems; London's residential areas grew to its west, with industry to the east so the wealthy could avoid downwind air pollution; health concerns led New York and many other US cities to create parks and gardens. Covid may yet change where people live and work in future.

But now we are seeing fast-growing cities affect human health on another scale as urban areas of more than 20 million people emerge and hundreds of smaller cities sprawl over wetlands and coasts, expand into forests and emit vast quantities of pollution. By 2100, there are likely to be many hundreds of cities far larger than Accra is today and the world's population centres will have shifted to Asia and Africa, with only a handful of the largest cities expected to be in Europe or North America.

I turned to David Satterthwaite, an urban expert at the International Institute for Environment and Development in London who has spent a lifetime observing the global population explosion and resultant growth of cities. 'What happens to cities over the next fifty years will transform both the global environment and the health of the eleven billion people expected to be alive then. The scale of urban population growth is astonishing. The fact is that much of humanity is young, fertile and increasingly urban. Delhi has grown by an average of 730,000 new residents a year for twenty years; Shanghai 641,000; Dhaka 536,000; Beijing 509,000; and São Paulo, with slower population growth rate, still adds a quarter of a million more persons a year.'

* * *

Lagos, like all megacities in tropical countries, is now a global reservoir of pathogens, its geography and connections to other cities making it prone to spreading infectious diseases. At one point in 2021 this one city simultaneously hosted the second largest HIV/Aids epidemic in the world, a linked TB epidemic and outbreaks of Lassa fever, Mpox, measles, yellow fever, swine fever and Covid-19.[2] Nowhere else could have coped and it is to its great credit that its massively overstretched public health service managed to contain them all, even stamping out more recent Zika and potential Ebola outbreaks. Unsurprisingly, it is frequently ranked one of the least liveable cities in the world.[3]

Even as Covid-19 was spreading through the city in 2021, Chikwe Ihekweazu, Nigeria's leading epidemiologist, and the World Health Organization's assistant director-general of health emergency intelligence tried to explain to me and the press how bad the health situation can be in a city like Lagos. 'Health is the greatest problem. There is no escape from disease outbreaks because of urbanisation and a lack of adequate water and sanitation. We battle with other infectious diseases. Every week, we detect cases of yellow fever, Lassa fever, measles and others. That is our reality – our tropical climate, urban population density, and poverty leave us at risk of annual, multiple, concurrent disease outbreaks.'[4]

Popular opinion suggests that African and Asian cities are unhealthy because of their lack of planning and infrastructure, but history shows that it was only when Europeans started to colonise countries that serious epidemics of flu, plague, malaria, cholera and waterborne diseases became common.[5]

Europeans visiting West Africa up to the nineteenth century had died in droves because they had poor immunity to tropical diseases,[6] but it was in the later nineteenth century, when colonial capital cities and ports were established and trade expanded, that huge numbers of local people were encouraged to come to them from the countryside for work. The result was predictable. The work camps were often built on marshy coastal land, and without sanitation, they became infested with rats and mosquitoes. The colonists took no responsibility for planning or health and these crowded places became the first slums, made worse because the many African colonies were linked by new shipping routes, so diseases like plague and flu were regularly passed along the African coast.[7]

I contacted prominent Nigerian urban historian Layi Egunjobi, director of the Centre for Urban and Regional Planning at Ibadan University, who described to me shortly before he died in 2016 how fast-growing colonial cities became progressively diseased. A pattern emerged, he said: 'The expanding cities created urban employment, which encouraged many young men to migrate alone from the interior to earn money. But with no help from the colonial powers or family to instruct them, the young men lived in squalor and waterborne diseases like cholera, typhoid and diarrhoea became inevitable in their camps.'[8]

As long ago as 29 November 1884, the *Nigeria Pioneer* newspaper noted the link between smallpox incidence and overcrowded slum housing in certain districts of Lagos. 'Within a few decades, both the new urban and the old natural environments were overwhelmed. As coastal forests were felled, mosquito-borne diseases like malaria and dengue emerged and European diseases like measles, mumps and tuberculosis arrived and spread from port to port and from community to community.'

In 1991 Egunjobi had vividly described the old core area of Lagos: 'The scene [was] one of overcrowding, lack of access roads, scarcity of drinking-water, ramshackle buildings, uncollected garbage, lack of sewers, inadequate air-space, and a housing environment littered with human faeces. All of these are conducive to the spread of tuberculosis, pneumonia, influenza, threadworm, cholera, dysentery and other diarrhoeal diseases.'[9]

* * *

When it came to disease, nowhere, I thought, compared to Lagos. But I was wrong. Dhaka, the fast-growing capital city of Bangladesh, was in another league altogether. Through British aid agency Oxfam I had met Mukta, a young woman, perhaps twenty years old, in an area of the city called Bari Badh. She and her family lived in a stilt house built over a lagoon. Behind it were blocks of fancy new flats and a busy main road.

But this was no prime real estate with a view. Dhaka was growing fast and Bari Badh was one of dozens of Dhaka shanty towns that displaced people had set up. Mukta's room was a windowless, two-square-metre shelter built of old bamboo, plastic, corrugated iron and cardboard, which she shared with five members of her family. They reached it by a wobbly, narrow walkway which stretched thirty metres over the water that swirled less than a metre below her bed. The latrine at the end of the walkway served more than a hundred people and was just a hole over the water screened by old hessian bags.

Built on the wrong side of a major river embankment, this slum took the brunt of the four-metre tidal surges and floods that sweep up from the Bay of Bengal and down the rivers. Mukta and her neighbours would now be called 'climate refugees' but fifteen years ago they were simply destitute. 'We were made homeless when our land was waterlogged. I knew that this was a risky place to live but we had no choice. There is a high risk of disease here, but where can I go?' she asked.

Her neighbour Firuza earned a pittance running a tea stall. Like many families in the city they too came from a coastal village which had been flooded again and again. In their short lives Firuza's children had suffered dysentery, typhoid and cholera. 'Many people here have jaundice. Everyone here has health problems. We used to beg clean water from the flats on the other side of the embankment. But people locked their doors and harassed us. So we took river water for boiling.'

Dhaka's slum dwellers are steadily being moved on because the land on which they live is often valuable. But new shanty towns appear as the city grows. Just thirty years ago this was a city of 250,000 people but it has mushroomed to 12 million and is growing by more than 1 million a year. Within ten years it is expected to have 23 million people, at least half of whom will be without basic services.

Lashed by summer monsoons, sited on a flood plain and surrounded by six great rivers, with another, the Buriganga, flowing through it, Dhaka is the capital of global disease, with its toxic air, polluted waters and slums. The Economist Intelligence Unit ranks it the second least 'liveable' in the world for its density of housing and congestion, but takes no account of its poverty and vulnerability to climate and quite ignores the fact that its people are some of the most welcoming and charming anywhere on earth.

When I was last there, a cholera epidemic had broken out even as dengue fever was spreading. I went to Outfall, another of many slums in the east of the city, to meet ten young women who had banded together to try to improve their own health and housing conditions. Vector-borne diseases like dengue and malaria were bad, of course, they said, but far worse were the everyday diseases their children caught from polluted water. We sat in a shack and I asked them if they knew of women whose children had died because of dirty water. There was a pause. Honufa shyly put her hand up. Then Taslima, then Rakhi. But they didn't just have second-hand experience, they said. Each of them said they had lost at least one child of their own. This was not unusual: 'Everyone gets ill here. We all have coughs, fevers and diarrhoeal diseases,' said Taslima.

I asked her friends if diseases were becoming more rife. 'Yes,' they all agreed.

Four child deaths between three women out of ten was not at all unusual, they said. Multiply Taslima, Honufa and Rakhi's experiences across the 500,000 or more other women living in city's slums, or the very many millions who lose their babies in Accra, Jakarta, Nairobi, Calcutta, Lima and a hundred other great developing world cities, and you can sense the heartbreak behind the cold health statistics which tell us that 2.4 billion people now live without sanitation, 1.2 billion do not have adequate water and 80 per cent of the world's illnesses are water-related.

We went outside. Taslima took my hand as she showed me an old hand pump drawing water from a shallow well about a hundred metres from her house. This, she said through an interpreter, was the source of many health problems. Her community suffered bouts of cholera, diarrhoea, dysentery and typhoid, typhus, schistosomiasis, river blindness, yellow fever and malaria. Shared by more than a thousand people, the well was an obvious health hazard, used by humans and animals, with rotting vegetable matter, puddles of stagnant water, mosquitoes, litter and even excreta. I asked why it could not be fixed. 'But it will cost $50. We do not have that,' was the reply.[10]

I gave the money and went on to see Azhurul Haq, then director of Dhaka's water authority. He may have had the most difficult job in the subcontinent. If Dhaka had been a city simply without money it would have been hard enough to keep it healthy. But, he told me, being built on a flood plain near the confluence of many large rivers, it regularly floods, sometimes so badly that tens of thousands of people must live for weeks in foul, polluted water and suffer a multitude of diseases.

He was honest but resigned:

This city is an incubator of disease, where all the conditions are met for outbreaks to occur. Who gets sick and where, depends only on where you live. The city has grown beyond belief with terrible results for health. The whole place is a landfill site and a cesspit. In some places, the waste is eight metres deep. We need a minimum of 1.6 billion litres of water a day. At the moment, our theoretical capacity is 1.35 billion litres a day and our actual production is 1.26 billion litres, which means that a lot of people cannot have clean water.

Preventing disease from the waste of 10 million people and some very polluting industries is even harder.

It is getting worse by the minute, not the day. Only 30 per cent of the city is covered by the sewerage system, and 90 per cent of it is untreated. We have sixteen lagoons where the waste goes, but people are cultivating fish in them and so the fish are loaded with heavy metals, too. There is a desperately serious problem of waterborne diseases here.

I thought I had seen the worst of disease in Asia, but I was wrong. In April 2017, just before the annual monsoon when the temperature was peaking at over 38°C and the humidity was suffocating, people in several districts started developing a fever, with rashes and severe muscle and joint pains. At first doctors thought it was dengue, another mosquito-borne disease which had flared up in the slums a month earlier, but within a few weeks it had spread to thousands of people and been identified as chikungunya, a mosquito-borne viral zoonotic disease identified for the first time in 1952 in Africa and only ever found twice before in rural Bangladesh. 'Chik', as it was known, raged for five months, in which time more than 13,000 people – possibly as many as twice that number – were infected. Chikungunya disappeared in September 2017 almost as unexpectedly as it had emerged. But there was no respite. Just eighteen months later, the city was devastated by its largest-ever outbreak of dengue fever. This time nearly 100,000 people were infected and several hundred died. When Covid-19 arrived in Dhaka in February 2020, it did not reach the poorest for several months, and then many thousands fled the city to return to their villages.[11] One year later there had officially been 684,756 cases and 9,739 deaths, almost certainly an undercount. I asked but no one could tell me what had happened to the women in Bari Badh and Outfall.

Even as I was visiting Bangladesh in 2014, the world's worst ever Ebola outbreak was ripping through the crowded slums of Monrovia, Freetown and Conakry in West Africa. The lethal disease that had until then been confined to villages and small populations in or near forests had exploded into these poor cities. For Robert Snyder and Claire Boone, two young epidemiologists at the UC Berkeley School of Health, it was deeply frustrating that the spotlight was on Western vaccines and laboratory research rather than on the elephant in the room – the slums where the disease was exploding and from which mutations will take place and pandemics will surely start.

They wrote to the *Lancet* saying that no one was paying any attention to the urban poor – the victims of a disease that could be contained: 'Ebola [is] just the beginning and only one disease; even if we are to control the current epidemic, the future introduction of this and other highly contagious and virulent microbes to and from global slums is inevitable.'[12]

One year later, Zika burst into the medical horror books with a viral strain causing malformation in infants whose mothers were infected during pregnancy. How it had evolved in the same mosquito that spread dengue and chikungunya viruses and reached the favelas of Rio and Recife by way of New Caledonia, the Cook Islands and Easter Island in the Pacific was still a mystery.

Once again Snyder and colleagues admonished governments for paying no attention to the urban poor where new diseases were continuing to explode, describing it as an 'act of hubris to think that a new vaccine, even if developed and shown to be effective … will successfully control this, or future epidemics of this virus that ravages urban slums'. They went on to add that resources 'must be harnessed and used to bring the largely ignored urban slum populations of megacities around the world into the global spotlight. Otherwise, we will continue to have the same inconsequential discussions until the next deadly epidemic is sparked in slums.'[13]

* * *

Neighbourhoods drowned and motorways became rivers when Hurricane Harvey dumped more than a metre of rain on Houston and parts of urban Texas in 2017. This was a result of climate change, it has been shown, but it came on top of disastrous urban planning, which is causing increasing numbers of disease outbreaks.

The Texas coastal climate is changing, the sea level is rising and there are more heavy downpours, Sam Brody, a Texas A&M University marine researcher who specialises in natural hazards told me. But he believed the addition of more than a million people moving to flood-prone areas near Houston since 2000 had overwhelmed the city's ability to drain water. 'If you are going to put 4 million people in this flood-vulnerable area in a way which involves ubiquitous application of impervious surfaces, you're going to get flooding. The driving force for the catastrophe was the built environment, the developers who paved over the wetlands, and the city authorities who gave them permission but who ignored the many warnings that flooding would follow.[14] The result was not only damage to infrastructure and deaths, but long-term mental health and stress problems, allergies and respiratory illness.'[15]

Similarly in South Asia, growth at breakneck speed has destroyed the ecology of cities, leading inevitably to floods and disease. I spoke with T. V. Ramachandra at the Indian Institute of Science, who was in despair about the health of the urban environment in Bangalore, now one of the world's fastest-growing IT centres. 'I loved this city. It was renowned for its trees and lakes and pleasant air. It was a truly healthy city. Now it's a dead city that has sacrificed its environment. Air pollution is at dangerous levels, the water is polluted, there is nowhere for the waste to go, and the lakes have been killed,' he said. 'People are moving out. Illnesses are increasing. At this rate every house will need a dialysis machine. Bangalore cannot continue like this. It is becoming an unlivable city. This is the worst city in the world for unchecked urbanisation,' he said.[16]

'Bangalore is typical of what is happening throughout India and China. It has tripled in size since 1995, the temperature in the city has risen between 2°C and 2.5°C and since 2000 it has flooded regularly. It is experiencing unprecedented, unrealistic and irresponsible urbanisation and sprawl. Most of the vegetation has been lost, 75 per cent of the city surface is impervious to water and the 2,500 lakes which used to store water have been drained for development,' said Ramachandra.

All ecological sense has been ditched, with profound consequences for health and the spread of disease, he continued. 'Cities have expanded into marshes, wetlands and flood-prone areas as populations have grown and people have moved from rural to urban areas in search of work. The result has been that the scale, intensity and duration of floods has increased and with them diseases. The diseases we see today are now man-made. They are not natural disasters. They are very similar and largely because of concretisation.'[17]

The health cost has been huge. India's air pollution is as bad as China's was in the 2000s, with 1.1 million people dying prematurely in 2015 alone from poor air quality linked to the hyper-development taking place in many cities.[18]

Urban researchers are now predicting that many of the world's largest cities can expect to be flooded as rapid urban expansions combine. Ramachandra says, 'When storms or floods hit cities, it is generally low-income groups that are hit hardest. Many informal settlements develop on land at high risk of flooding or landslides because their inhabitants cannot afford safer sites.'[19]

Flooding is already one of the world's greatest causes of illness and death. According to the Flood Observatory at Dartmouth College, urban sprawl may be just as much to blame for floods as climate change. Researchers there collated global media reports and found that between 1985 and 2014 floods worldwide killed more than 500,000 people, displaced over 650 million people and caused $800 billion worth of damage. Between 2003 and 2008 alone, large-scale floods occurred in more than 1,800 cities in forty countries.[20]

* * *

I wanted to nail down the links between population growth and the emergence of diseases. I had been urged to visit Naa Puowele Karbo, Paramount Chief of Lawra, an area in the far north of Ghana, who had spent his life trying to control the tide of young people leaving the countryside for the cities and to improve urban health. Under his watch as director of planning, Accra, the capital, had grown from a small town the size of Shrewsbury to a city of over 6 million people in just thirty years.

With Jerry Sam, a young Accravian, I flew to Tamale, Ghana's third-largest city, hired an old banger and a driver and drove the last 300 kilometres along some of the worst roads in Africa, passing the great Bole National Park with its elephants and baboons and villages with names such as Tuna and Ya, and shops called The Forgive and Forget Chemical Drug Store. Late in the evening we presented ourselves at the palace in Lawra, a rambling collection of low buildings, some built underground, a courtyard dominated by two enormous marble graves and several flagpoles. We were greeted by the chief's brother, who said he knew we were coming because our car made an unusual sound. We arranged to meet the family the next day.

'First,' said Puowele, when we met, 'you must understand that the concept of children in rural Africa sixty years ago was very different. Children in those days defined men's social standing, they were needed to increase wealth, they were assets to work the fields and fetch water, but numbers did not matter. A man did not look after them, and no one actually knew how big families were.'

His own father, King Karbo I, had seemingly been on a mission to populate Ghana single-handed. When he died in 1967, the family tried to count his offspring. 'I did a population census of him in 1970. We counted about seventy daughters and thirty-five sons. He left thirty-nine widows. I could not count them all. Our children are many, and traditionally we don't count them. We don't actually know how many he had – he never counted them. He tried keeping records, but it didn't work.'

Today, said Puowele, children are no longer seen as an asset. 'The trend is downwards. Nowadays the demands [on families] are great. You are in deep shit if you have too many. So you go for quality rather than numbers.'

But it was not for want of knowledge so much as deliberate neglect and the policy of rich countries that health in Ghana and across much of Africa had deteriorated, he said.

Cities like Accra are undoubtedly a mess with a massive health problem. We had drawn up plans, and knew exactly what was needed to avoid infectious diseases catching hold and spreading. But the rich countries like Britain and the US refused to help financially, and the World Bank, IMF and global finance groups forced Ghana and other countries to open their markets to promote growth and did not allow them to spend money on health or education. That is why Africa and so many other parts of the world now know so much disease and why epidemics are so likely to occur.

[Because of this] we just could not control the population or the health of the city. We created a green belt, we planned reservoirs to stop flooding, we planned for oil, we knew what to do but the [politicians] refused to implement these things and there was no money.

He and his colleagues even considered building a healthy new capital city to take pressure off Accra.

We looked at Abuja, the purpose-built capital of Nigeria. You can build a city from scratch, but if you do not change behaviour, it will be the same as the old one. Now we are approaching our ecological limits. Our environment has suffered badly from the pressure of numbers, our natural resources are diminishing. Our forests are being cut down. We can no longer find the herbs we used to use. Climate change is taking place.

But the future was not bleak, he told me. Like most Ghanaians, he believed that, if planned better and given a fair wind and a political will, Africa's burgeoning population will be the key to its future prosperity and its health. 'We will have to diversify, yes. We will learn new things. But we are still confident in the future.'

PART III

THE WAYS AHEAD

We need the tonic of wildness … we can never have enough of nature.

Henry David Thoreau, *Walden*, 1854

14

THE NEXT PANDEMIC

When he bought the pretty little striped field mouse on the internet for $8 to give to his daughter for her sixth birthday, the businessman from São Paulo in Brazil was told it had been bred by a registered dealer. In fact, it had been sourced from the vast upstate sugar cane fields that had been planted recently to grow biofuels to reduce the use of fossil fuels, and which were swarming with rodents after another heatwave.

Two days later it bit his daughter on the finger but neither she nor he thought much of it. Ten days later he left on a business trip to Europe. By the time he reached Amsterdam his daughter had started suffering fevers, muscle aches and breathing problems and been rushed to hospital, and he, too, was unwell. After three nights feeling steadily worse in a hotel he went to the city's main teaching hospital. But it was too late. Unwittingly he had already passed the disease to several other people on the plane and a chambermaid at his hotel. It was the start of the worst pandemic of modern times, ruining countries and killing and infecting far more people than Covid-19 had done.

The first small 'outbreaks of unknown origin' were posted on ProMed, a website for reporting global daily infectious disease outbreaks, and both Dutch and Brazilian virologists soon identified a respiratory hantavirus, a group of lethal diseases transmitted by rodents. But this was unlike any other hantavirus they had seen: it was a genetically new and distinct virus that had evidently adapted to its new environment in the cane fields and was able to evade all known vaccines and attack people of all ages. No vaccines or drugs were available.

Within two weeks a hundred people on two continents were infected and forty people had died. Soon numbers were doubling every few days and it was detected in thirty countries. But while Covid-19 had killed about 1 per cent of the people it infected, this hantavirus had a mortality rate of nearly 50 per cent – as severe as Ebola – and it seemed to be able to spread as fast as the Omicron variant of Covid-19.

The WHO declared a pandemic just before the number of cases exploded and warned governments to expect waves of infection. This was Covid-19 on steroids and it was dubbed by journalists 'Disease X', the name given by the WHO years before to a hypothetical pathogen so transmissible and lethal that it could potentially kill hundreds of millions of people before any vaccine or cure had been developed or distributed in large numbers.

Disease X struck with unimaginable speed and ferocity. It moved wherever people moved. It ripped through the great crowded cities of Africa, Latin America and Southeast Asia and then rich cities like Los Angeles, Paris and London. Like Covid-19, the plague and every other pandemic, it preyed on the inequalities in societies and spared no one.

Now the real panic started. Most people never stood a chance. Borders were slammed shut and lockdowns imposed on angry communities, as governments rushed to find, isolate and trace victims. Epidemiologists knew that if it continued to spread this fast, it would overwhelm health systems, morgues and governments in a few months. Scientists and governments raced to design, test, license, make and then distribute effective vaccines, but it still took six months to rush them out, by which time 70 million people had been infected and 20 million had died. As with Covid-19 in 2020, there was opposition, but this time there were also food shortages and riots, economic chaos and political turmoil.

Back in 2020 it had surprised people that an invisible microbe could jump from a bat or a pangolin to a human and cause so much damage. But Covid-19 had been all but forgotten and this time no one thought that a mouse belonging to a six-year-old child could result in 200 million deaths and 1 billion infections, far more than had died in a hundred years of war and four times as many as had died in the 1918 Spanish flu pandemic – until then, the worst the modern world had known.

* * *

Disease X is hypothetical but it is surely coming. It may not be a hantavirus, and it may not arrive for many decades, but with climate change and new ecological conditions in so many places and dense human and animal populations, the prospect of more deadly, more frequent and, possibly, simultaneous disease outbreaks becomes inevitable. The next great pandemic could just as well be a bird flu, a coronavirus like Covid-19 or a souped-up ancient killer like typhoid or plague. It may spill over to humans via a hamster, a bat, a chicken, a tick or a reptile. It could spread from a hospital ward with a fungal disease that resists antimicrobial drugs, or come out of a fur farm in Norway or a chicken megafarm in Nigeria. It could just as easily incubate in a forest or a lab.

The term 'Disease X' is thought to have been coined by Stanford University virologist Nathan Wolfe, then adopted by scientists at the World Health assembly in Geneva in 2017 and first used by the WHO in 2018. Disease experts crossing wildlife and human disease disciplines were asked to draw up a priority list of pathogens thought to represent the most serious threats to global health. They judged some diseases to be particularly dangerous because they were so lethal, others because they could spread extremely fast, and some because the environmental conditions were just right for them to emerge from degraded forests, intensive farms, urban slums or animal markets. Their final list included HIV/Aids, Ebola, SARS, avian flus, Zika and MERS. But they added 'Disease X' to suggest that some unknown pathogen for which no drugs or vaccines were yet in the pipeline could emerge to kill hundreds of millions of people.

One of the scientists in Geneva was Edinburgh University epidemiologist Mark Woolhouse. During the Covid-19 crisis he explained to me why they gave a name to a non-existent disease:

> We thought that the next emerging pandemic might be a virus
> that we don't even know about yet – quite frankly we thought
> it was the most likely scenario. Every year, two or three new
> viruses that are transmissible to humans are found, and the rate
> has been constant for more than fifty years. There is a lot of
> discussion about how many potential Disease Xs are out there,
> but no one thinks we have finished discovering them. It is a
> matter of when the next pandemic will hit, not if.[1]

Another scientist at the 2017 Geneva meeting was Peter Daszak, the British zoologist who had co-founded the US-based EcoHealth alliance, a collection of disease and wildlife experts working in China and elsewhere to identify viruses and head off future pandemics. '[They] should be treated like terrorist attacks,' he said, 'because governments know roughly where they originate and what is responsible for them, but do not know when the next one will happen.' He wrote about Disease X in 2020: 'We said back then, in Geneva [that it] would likely result from a virus originating in animals and would emerge somewhere on the planet where economic development drives people and wildlife together. [It] would probably be confused with other diseases early in the outbreak and would spread quickly and silently; exploiting networks of human travel and trade, it would reach multiple countries and thwart containment. Disease X would have a mortality rate higher than a seasonal flu but would spread as easily as the flu. It would shake financial markets even before it achieved pandemic status.'[2]

The facts are stark. There have been six influenza pandemics in just over a century, which have together killed more than 60 million people and infected several billion people. HIV/Aids has so far killed around 38 million people and continues to infect 37 million each year. Ebola, one of the most dangerous diseases the world has ever known, has spilled over from animals about twenty-five times in fifty years, and at least seven coronaviruses, including Covid-19, have brought illness and death to hundreds of millions of people. In just the last decade we have had a major outbreak of Ebola, which killed thousands of people but, almost miraculously, did not spread around the world, as well as a significant outbreak of Zika in Latin America.

Some 500 new zoonotic diseases have been detected since the 1950s and any one of them could theoretically have turned into a pandemic. 'Every century has had its Disease X,' says Canadian medical historian Tom Koch. 'Plague devastated Europe in the fourteenth and fifteenth centuries, yellow fever hit the Americas in the eighteenth century and cholera was the global threat in the nineteenth century. In the past hundred years SARS, MERS, influenza, Ebola, Marburg, Lassa, Nipah, Zika and now Covid-19 each have been the Disease X of their time.'

All pandemics, Koch told me, are evidence of rapid evolution in the microbial world, which is what the world is seeing now. 'We should expect virulent new diseases to emerge and new pandemics to spread. Old diseases like tuberculosis are returning in new and more virulent forms and newly evolved bacteria and viruses are at the same time appearing. Our microbial friends are evolving and we are not. The best of science will not be effective against a rapidly evolving bacterium or virus.'[3]

Koch argues that the way we live today is causing new diseases to emerge and old ones to acquire new traits. 'We are pushing the evolutionary advance of microbes in any number of ways and then are surprised when they respond. We have seen new infections spread globally for centuries. What we are now experiencing is the bill coming due, as deforestation, industrialisation, urbanisation and income inequality pressure the ecologies in which we and those microbes together exist. When the next pandemic will come and what it will be, nobody knows. But we know there will be one. And given the increased rate of epidemic outbreaks from a range of bacteria and viruses probably in the next five to eight years,' he told Paul Gallagher, the *I*'s health correspondent.[4]

* * *

All the planetary conditions for Disease X to emerge and spread rapidly through a hot, crowded world are now in place. Climate change is shifting the range of animals and their pathogens; forests are being cut down to make way for pasture and palm plantations, making it more likely that pathogens will emerge; mutations and reassortments of viruses are taking place regularly in poultry farms; and people are travelling further and faster than ever before. Disease X could be spread by the boot of a pilgrim on Haj, the tyre of a lorry carrying animal feed to a pig farm in Ukraine, a migrant from Central America or a mosquito hitching a ride on a cargo ship from China to Fiji. We just do not know.

Pandemics today are not just man-made, but inevitable, says Daszak. 'They are [happening] more like once every ten years right now and they are getting more frequent and damaging. It is the same human activities that drive climate change and biodiversity that drive pandemic risk through their impacts on our environment. Changes in the way we use land; the expansion and intensification of agriculture; and unsustainable trade, production and consumption disrupt nature and increase contact between wildlife, livestock, pathogens and people. We can escape the era of pandemics, but this requires a much greater focus on prevention, in addition to reaction.'[5]

Other infectious disease physicians offer similar predictions. Anthony Fauci, veteran director of the US National Institute of Allergy and Infectious Diseases, writing with colleague David Morens in the journal *Cell*, put it like this:

As human societies grow in size and complexity, we create an endless variety of opportunities for genetically unstable infectious agents to emerge into the unfilled ecological niches we continue to create. There is nothing new about this situation, except that we now live in a human-dominated world in which our increasingly extreme alterations of the environment induce increasingly extreme backlashes from nature.[6]

Virologist and NIH flu expert David Morens adds that pandemics should be treated on the same danger level as nuclear war. 'Today, we have international agencies, treaties, and agreements dedicated to preventing nuclear wars. Scientific evidence – and our collective daily experience coping with Covid-19 – tells us that pandemics may equal or surpass the effects of terrorism or a nuclear attack. It is time to significantly elevate our response to them so it is equal to the peril they present.'[7]

In the last few years, the trickle of leading scientists who have argued that pandemics are rooted in the human destruction of the global environment has become a river and is now a flood. 'There is a single species responsible for the Covid-19 pandemic – us,' said professors Josef Settele, Sandra Díaz and Eduardo Brondizio, who led a global report into the links between biodiversity and disease: 'Recent pandemics are a direct consequence of human activity, particularly our global financial and economic systems that prize economic growth at any cost.'[8]

When Covid-19 struck, I talked to legendary biologist Thomas Lovejoy, one of the giants of global conservation who coined the term 'biodiversity' and founded an extraordinary education project in the heart of the Amazon. 'We humans did this [Covid-19] to ourselves. This was our disease. A new pandemic to which we have no immunity will emerge within a few years.'[9] He himself died in December 2021 as US deaths from Covid-19 passed 850,000 and showed no signs of stopping.

* * *

Just how serious the situation is can be seen in the trends of human, animal and plant health. Individually many show accelerating rises in disease levels, but together they suggest that all areas of human, wild and farmed life are increasingly diseased. The number of human disease outbreaks, the number of diseases involved in these outbreaks and the number of countries affected by these outbreaks have all grown in the last forty years.[10] Meanwhile the individual outbreaks have become increasingly pandemic, or widespread.[11] In just seven years, the US Centers for Disease Control recognised 1,485 epidemics of more than forty human diseases in 172 countries – far more than had been recognised in the previous thirty years.[12]

What about animal disease outbreaks? Over roughly the same period of time, the World Organisation for Animal Health (OIE) reported growing numbers of cattle, poultry and pig disease outbreaks.[13] In 2021 alone, forty-one countries on three continents had widespread cases of avian flu in poultry, and African swine fever had swept through the world's pig farms. Human infections were low, but at least two avian flu subtypes, H5N6 and H5N1, were now a 'serious threat to [human] health. By December 2021, Covid-19 had also been documented in domestic cats and dogs, ferrets, bats, mink, primates, pangolins, pigs, rodents and deer.[14]

It was the same with plants. IPBES, the UN's monitor of trends in the natural world, reported in 2019 that humans were driving 1 million species to extinction,[15] and the UN's agriculture body, the Food and Agriculture Organization, said that outbreaks of crop and forest insect pests and diseases were also on the increase globally.[16]

Covid-19 is far from alone as an active epidemic. I chose at random April 2022 to check what other major infectious diseases, mostly passed to humans from animals, were emerging or ongoing. The ProMed website, used by epidemiologists to alert each other and governments, showed a new surge of Ebola in Congo, Lassa fever and Mpox in Nigeria and anthrax in Argentina, as well as outbreaks of leprosy, polio, yellow fever, meningitis, plague, dengue, Zika, chikungunya, Kyasanur Forest disease and other mosquito-borne diseases in many places. Measles and cholera were making comebacks; rabies was rife in Mexico and typhoid in Fiji. One study of game animals commonly eaten in China identified seventy-one mammal viruses circulating, including eighteen deemed of potentially high risk to both people and domestic animals.[17] Adding to the list of more than thirty human infectious diseases that month were major outbreaks of viral diseases in many fruit and grain crops and ongoing pandemic diseases in cattle, birds, deer, sheep and pigs.

The fact that all these diseases had been notified in that one month suggests surveillance was working, but what alarms epidemiologists is that many outbreaks are of diseases either new to science or much older ones re-emerging in more virulent form. They include five new pandemic influenza variants linked to intensive poultry and pork production; half a dozen exotic or hemorrhagic diseases like Ebola, Nipah and Hendra, linked to bats and habitat destruction, and several transmitted by mosquitoes and ticks, which have greatly extended their ranges, probably because of global heating and changing environmental conditions.

Nearly three-quarters of the 1,485 outbreaks identified by the US Centers for Disease Control were zoonotic in origin and at least eighteen diseases, like plague, cholera, typhoid and yellow fever, had been known for hundreds of years but had re-emerged, sometimes in a deadlier or more transmissible form than before. Most had killed just a few hundred people before fizzling out, but one, HIV/Aids, has so far killed more than 20 million people worldwide and is far from over. Covid-19 was not included in the report; nor were non-communicable diseases like asthma triggered by air pollution.

The human cost of death and disease is incalculable, but the economic cost can be roughly measured. If Covid-19 is included, diseases in humans may have cost $11 trillion – more than the top fifteen countries spent on armaments in 2020 in just seven years,[18] and far more than the $7.8 trillion spent worldwide on health in 2017. If pandemics of animal diseases like bird flu and African swine fever are included, the cost rises by hundreds of millions more dollars.[19] If the reduced crops, diseased animal herds, human hunger and loss of biodiversity linked to man-made climate change were factored in, we would have to conclude that we live in a very sick world.

* * *

Pandemics always take countries by surprise. In November 2013 a previously healthy retired Saudi soldier was admitted to the intensive care unit of the King Abdulaziz University Hospital in

Jeddah with a fever. Two weeks later, severely short of breath and with his organs failing, he died.[20] Researchers quickly identified the cause. The sixty-year-old man had been breeding dromedary camels in a shed, and nursing closely one that was ill. A nose swab showed that they were both infected with a highly pathogenic coronavirus called Middle East respiratory syndrome, or MERS.

Camel milk is now a multi-million dollar a year industry and it was known that MERS circulated harmlessly but widely in the animal population. Nearly half of Kenya's 3 million or more camels had already been exposed to MERS,[21] along with many of their handlers, but alarm bells rang when it was found that the disease could also be transmitted from humans to humans. Soon, other human cases of MERS, not connected to camels, were appearing in Spain, the UAE, South Korea and elsewhere. Pilgrims on Haj, the annual Muslim pilgrimage to Mecca in Saudi Arabia, were warned to avoid contact with camels and the Middle East's many camel farmers were informed.

Like SARS before it, and Covid-19 in 2019, MERS came from the large family of coronaviruses and, also like them, probably emerged from bats, which made camels their reservoir host. It was just the latest shot in a barrage of unexpected diseases to spill over from animals and strike in the early 2000s. In the decade since it made the jump to humans it has killed nearly 2,500 people in twenty-seven countries, hit some economies hard and threatened to mutate, possibly into something less deadly but more easily transmissible.[22]

Happily, earlier work done to develop vaccines against it and SARS gave scientists like Sarah Gilbert at the Jenner Institute in Oxford an advantage in the global race to develop a vaccine when Covid-19 emerged. When MERS had first jumped to humans, Gilbert had travelled to Saudi Arabia to study the disease. Over the next few years, working in Oxford with mice, she and others established the virus's biology, how it behaved and its weak spots. Within months of Covid-19's outbreak in China they had developed a vaccine but without their earlier work on MERS. it would almost certainly have taken longer to develop and millions more people would have probably been hospitalised. It was the camel, it might be said, which broke the back of Covid-19.

Yet no one had expected that MERS would jump to humans. Like HIV/Aids in the 1980s, and then Ebola, Nipah and SARS, it came out of the blue and no one knows to this day exactly why it emerged in Saudi Arabia just then. Indeed, it could have been circulating quietly for years. '[It] took the world by surprise. No one's eye was on camels in the Middle East. We were thinking something flu-like from Southeast Asia or Africa,' Delia Grace Randolph, co-leader of animal and human health at the International Livestock Research Institute in Nairobi, Kenya told me.[23]

The consensus now is that MERS was effectively man-made, another result of people farming animals intensively and unnaturally, in this case packed in sheds without safeguards – the perfect conditions for a disease to emerge and jump, or spill over, to humans. 'Camels used to always be kept free-range. They have become very valuable in the Middle East with oil money, but instead of being farmed free-range … they were being put in sheds. Lots of camels together leads to more contact between them and more camel-to-human contact. When you change a farming system, you run risks,' said Randolph.[24]

She expects the world to get a wave of new zoonotic diseases, a mixture of old and new ones, but when and where they emerge it will be hard to know. 'Animals have thousands of viruses. These will continue to emerge in predictably unpredictable ways and places. But others will certainly emerge which we did not know about. The worst may be yet to come.'

In evolutionary terms, virologists often say, we are experiencing microbial turmoil. All species share pathogens all the time and it is through this process that life mutates and evolves. But until now the process of species mutating, thriving, declining and eventually dying out has been slow, taking place over millennia. What is changing is the speed of the changes and the balance of nature. It is from this microbial chaos that disease emerges.

Only in the past fifty years has humanity's impact on the planet been widely understood, and it's taken even less time for it to be known that most diseases are being driven by human behaviour. In just five centuries, less than the blink of an eye in evolutionary terms, humankind has become so ecologically dominant that it has changed the geography of life and created the conditions for diseases to emerge and spread. Instead of thinking of pandemics, whether of plants, animals or people, as rare events, we should think of them as the coming normal.

It may take an infinite number of chance encounters for a virus to evolve to successfully jump between species, but by disturbing the environment so dramatically and so fast, humans are increasing the likelihood of spillovers. Fast-growing human and farmed animal populations throw pathogens closer together than ever before; the more mouths there are to feed, the more agriculture and cities must expand; our technologies have enabled the quick and easy transport of pathogens around the world and our economic system has led to the exponential expansion of trade; our warming of the earth's atmosphere and pollution of the land and seas puts increased pressure on other species' habitats and so drives the spillover of pathogens from one species to another.

It's now a numbers game, says Rick Ostfeld, a disease ecologist at the Cary Institute of Ecosystem Studies in Millbrook, New York, who with Felicia Keesing has done so much to show how human disease and biodiversity are linked:

When we erode biodiversity, we favour species that are more likely to become zoonotic hosts. There is a widespread misconception that wild nature is the greatest source of zoonotic disease. This idea is reinforced by popular culture portrayals of jungles teeming with microbial menaces. The great zoonotic threats actually arise where natural areas have been converted to cropland, pastures and urban areas. The next pandemic disease is far more likely to come from a rat than a rhino. We inadvertently make life golden for the rats of the world by replacing native habitat with strip malls, megadams and soybean fields.[25]

The message is stark but starting to get through to politicians. In an open letter to President Biden imploring the US government to prepare now for the next pandemic, Mitch McConnell and other US senators said: 'With six times more outbreaks in 2010 than 1980, the next million-death pandemic is more likely to happen in the next decade than in the next century and will almost certainly be the result of another zoonotic spillover.'[26]

Consensus is growing that the risk of emerging zoonotic diseases is greatest where humans disturb natural environments the most. Raina Plowright, a wildlife vet leading a team of seventy disease ecologists investigating how bats pass coronaviruses and other pathogens to humans, sums up the situation we find ourselves in:

> As we fragment landscapes, we ... need to understand that human health is an ecological service. It's a service that nature is providing us, so we need to protect nature to protect ourselves. We are playing a Ponzi scheme with the ecosystems that allow our planet to survive.[27]

GREAT ESCAPES

Janet Parker woke on a beautiful 1978 summer morning in a leafy Birmingham, UK, suburb to find she had a skin rash and a few flat, red spots on her face. She dismissed it as a flu, stayed in bed and thought little more of it. But two days later she had excruciating headaches and the spots had spread to her torso, legs and feet. Then the high fevers and sore throat began.

The kindly, middle-aged photographer was worried enough to call her doctor, who thought it was chickenpox but to be safe sent her to the local hospital, thereby probably avoiding a pandemic of an ancient disease that in the course of 3,000 years had killed possibly 500 million people, including Egyptian pharaohs and French kings.[1]

Janet Parker had smallpox. She had caught it from the university laboratory of the distinguished British virologist Henry Bedson, which she sometimes visited. As soon as it was confirmed, a massive effort was mounted to stop the disease spreading. Smallpox kills 15–30 per cent of people it touches, and those it spares are often left blind or horribly scarred.

After two weeks in hospital she was hanging on to life. Her face was described as being a 'reddish hue … [with] a sorry, sad, exhausted look of resignation'. But she was not the first to die. On 1 September 1978, harassed by the press, appalled by the disrepute into which he felt he had dragged his family and unable to comprehend how the disease could have escaped from his laboratory, Henry

Bedson cut his throat in a garden shed. Janet Parker died ten days later at 3.50 a.m., the last person in the world known to have been killed by smallpox.

Her death brought to light dozens of other laboratory accidents, all marked by carelessness, defective equipment or human error. A similar smallpox outbreak in 1966 had seen another medical photographer working at the same Birmingham medical school contract a mild form of the disease and in 1972 two researchers watching the harvesting of live smallpox virus from eggs at a laboratory in the London School of Hygiene and Tropical Medicine were infected and also died. It was easier to catch smallpox in Britain, it seemed, than in Africa.

The risk of a pandemic starting in a laboratory grows every year despite rigorous safety procedures and ever-tighter rules and protocols. Medical and military research uses the world's most dangerous bacteria, viruses and pathogens and is now conducted in thousands of state, corporate and academic laboratories around the world. New ways to find vaccines and control dangerous pathogens are now a multi-billion-dollar global industry employing tens of thousands of people.

Veteran researcher Lynn Klotz at the Washington-based US Center for Arms Control and Non-Proliferation is convinced there is a 'substantial probability' that a pandemic with over 100 million deaths could be seeded from the laboratory escape of a pathogen. The historical record, he says, reveals labs to be the cause of at least one global flu pandemic, several smallpox escapes, major foot and mouth epidemics, a SARS outbreak and hundreds more smaller but potentially lethal escapes from labs in the US, Russia, UK and elsewhere.[2]

Over time, lab accidents will always happen, he says. Job stress, carelessness, failures in procedures, pipette spills, needle pricks in safety suits, lack of training and slack safety cultures all can and do lead to accidents. Protective clothing can tear, vials of viruses and bacteria can go missing or break in transit, technicians can be bitten by infected animals.[3] Lab waste, too, can contain viruses, bacteria or microbes and deadly pathogens have even been sent to the wrong address.[4]

Klotz has uncovered appalling biosafety conditions. After one accident in a high-level laboratory at Erasmus University in the Netherlands, a worker who had been potentially exposed to a pandemic influenza virus was sent to quarantine at home. In another incident, a researcher was found to be wearing shorts when a spill of avian flu occurred. 'There is widespread evidence that even the world's most secure laboratories have been the source of disease outbreaks, accidents and possibly two pandemics.'[5] An explosion in the number of laboratories researching dangerous pathogens and potentially dangerous new technologies which enable researchers to make new viruses is leading to more close shaves and accidents, he fears.

His data, gleaned largely from US government institutions, suggests that more than 70 per cent of accidents are caused by human error. 'With just a few dozen laboratories studying potential pandemic pathogens there is an 80 per cent chance [one] will accidentally escape from at least one lab in a mere 12.8 years, an interval far shorter than those between natural flu pandemics in the twentieth century,' Klotz says. 'I am gravely concerned. The probability of a lab incident or accident is much too high.'[6]

Just getting reliable information on escapes is tortuous, says Israel Institute of Technology researcher David Manheim. Data is not made public, records are not always kept, scientists and universities are reluctant to admit errors, government agencies are by habit secretive and scientists fear for their jobs. The very great majority of incidents known about are contained quickly and no harm is done but he has documented seventy-one major incidents involving accidental or deliberate exposures of highly pathogenic agents since 1976. They include researchers dying of plague, cattle diseases, anthrax and salmonella, as well as from unknown pathogens. And that is not counting any military accidents. 'It is near certain that accidents involving biological weapons are, and will remain, unknown, if only because they would be illegal or constitute war crimes,' he says.[7]

* * *

Bio-containment labs are given Biological Safety Levels (BSLs) between 1 and 4. The lowest level, where pathogens not known to cause disease in humans are worked on, is quite basic. There must only be a lockable door, people must wash their hands when going in and out, and no food or drink is allowed in. Level 2 labs, where viruses causing diseases like hepatitis A, B and C, HIV/Aids and salmonella are handled, requires people to wear double gloves and face coverings and be trained.

Level 3 labs are a major step up. This is where the most potentially dangerous genetically modified organisms and viruses like West Nile, SARS, MERS, Rift Valley fever and yellow fever are handled. There are thought to be at least 200 of these labs in the US alone and similar numbers in the EU and elsewhere. They must be sealable and the air in them has to be filtered. To get in, you must shower and wear protective clothing, then pass through two sets of self-closing doors.

Level 4 labs are effectively bunkers within bunkers, used to diagnose infections with lethal and highly transmissible pathogens, and to conduct experiments where pathogens are genetically enhanced or manipulated for research. There are thought to be fewer than sixty of them worldwide and just to get into them, people need to be trained and to wear full body protective suits with their own independent air supply. They are mostly state-owned, sited in urban centres, and the work done in them is usually secret and often conducted for the military. The US has at least nine Level 4 labs, and numbers worldwide have grown as new techniques emerge to research pathogens for medical and military purposes. More countries are expected to seek BSL4 labs, too, in the wake of the Covid-19 pandemic as they seek to identify viruses which pose a higher risk of jumping from animals to humans or becoming transmissible between humans.

I was declined an interview three times with anyone at the UK's Ministry of Defence Porton Down bioweapons establishment in Wiltshire where most research is conducted into dangerous virus and pathogens. But I spoke to Filippa Lentzos, a biosecurity expert in the departments of War Studies and Global Health and Social

Medicine at King's College London. Human error, even in high-security laboratories that handle the most dangerous pathogens, must be taken seriously when assessing potential future pandemics, she said.

> Lab design cannot overcome human error or poor training.
> It's fairly rare to have accidents, but they happen all the time.
> They can result from a laboratory culture or an individual.
> Most researchers are working with pathogens with low
> epidemic potential, so there is no great risk. But others are
> highly dangerous. The risk of future pandemics originating
> from research with dangerous pathogens is real. The vast
> majority of countries with maximum containment labs do not
> regulate dual-use research, which refers to experiments that
> are conducted for peaceful purposes but can be adapted to
> cause harm; or gain-of-function research, which is focused on
> increasing the ability of a pathogen to cause disease. A large
> proportion of scientific research on coronaviruses is carried out
> in countries with no oversight of dual-use research or gain-of-
> function experiments.[8]

* * *

The heyday of known lab escapes was in the 1960s and '70s, when many new infectious diseases were emerging and safety was notoriously lax. Researcher Robert Pike at University of Texas Southwestern Medical Center in Dallas found official records in 1976 of an astonishing 3,921 'laboratory acquired infections' (LAIs) involving pathogens and animals, resulting in 164 deaths worldwide.[9] Marburg virus, similar to Ebola, was named after the small German town where, in 1967, twenty-five technicians in a vaccine lab were exposed to it from monkeys shipped there from Uganda. Thirty-one people who had contact with the blood, organs or cell cultures of the animals fell ill.

But pathogens have never stopped escaping. A study of US government reports found more than 1,100 lab incidents involving bacteria, viruses and toxins that pose 'significant or bioterror risks' between 2008 and 2012. A cursory search on the CDC website yields hundreds more.[10] According to the CDC and other databases, around half of all accidents and escapes require some sort of medical treatment. The greatest number appear to be in animal labs handling brucellosis. These are followed by TB and viruses transmitted by mosquitoes, like yellow fever, Zika and dengue fever.[11] Other accidents lead to salmonella, HIV and hantaviruses carried by rodents.[12]

Some escapes involve very dangerous pathogens. Russian researchers are also known to have been infected with Marburg fever; five Chinese technicians reportedly died during SARS experiments; polio, hepatitis C and Mpox have all escaped from vaccine labs, and plague was caught by a wildlife biologist and one scientist was exposed to Ebola.[13] Worryingly, the databases record more than 700 incidents of theft, loss and accidental releases of potentially lethal biological agents.[14]

A 2015 *USA Today* investigation found that more than a hundred US Level 3 and 4 labs handling the most dangerous pathogens had experienced the most egregious safety or security breaches. From 2006 to 2013, labs had notified federal regulators of about 1,100 incidents with nearly fifty 'select agent pathogens' deemed to pose bioterror threats. In more than 800 cases, workers had to receive medical treatment.[15] Of these, twenty-two people had to be treated for anthrax at a US military base.

The year 2014 was particularly bad, with the US CDC having to shut down two of its high-level biosafety labs and stop all transfers of samples.[16] A government scientist cleaning out a cold room between two labs at the National Institutes of Health in Bethesda, Maryland, opened a cardboard box and found decades-old vials of smallpox – years after all stocks were supposed to have been destroyed.[17] This was followed by seventy-five CDC workers being potentially exposed to anthrax when samples thought to be dead proved to be alive;[18] that same year a CDC laboratory sent a shipment of H9N2 avian influenza to a government poultry lab. As if that was not enough, a Chicago hospital worker picked up a fatal dose of plague in a laboratory, the US Army mistakenly sent live anthrax bacteria to nearly 200 labs around the world and the CDC sent the wrong batch of Ebola samples from a BSL4 lab to a less secure one.[19]

* * *

Meanwhile, the UK authorities have reported that public and private lab accidents involving dangerous bacteria, fungi and viruses are occurring regularly. *Guardian* science editor Ian Sample reported in 2014 how a schoolboy-level blunder led to live anthrax being sent by mistake from a government lab to dozens of others without warning.[20] Another error led to the escape of dengue virus, which kills 20,000 people worldwide each year – it was also posted by mistake. On one occasion students at the University of the West of England unwittingly studied live meningitis-causing germs which they thought had been killed by heat treatment. Inspections revealed torn isolation suits at a lab handling animals infected with Ebola, and a faulty air handling system at another lab handling foot and mouth.

Most releases are caught immediately and little harm is done. But sometimes the escapes threaten human or animal life on a large scale. In 2007, just six years after a catastrophic foot and mouth disease epidemic broke out in northern England, forcing the slaughter of 6 million cattle and sheep, another outbreak occurred, this time on a farm close to the UK's government animal health laboratories at Pirbright.[21] Investigators quickly identified it as a strain not naturally found in the environment and traced its release to a cracked pipe linking the government's Institute of Animal Health and two pharmaceutical companies, both of which had laboratories on the site. Another bullet had been dodged but eight farms were infected and 1,578 animals had to be slaughtered.

Some mistakes are so stupid as to be barely comprehensible. In 2005 the virus that caused the massive 1957 Asian flu pandemic was accidentally released by a lab in the US and sent all over the world in 3,700 test kits. The mistake was discovered only after the virus escaped at a high-containment lab in Canada. The kits should have contained a particular strain of influenza A – the viral family that causes most flu worldwide. But the contractors somehow chose the 1957 pandemic strain. Thankfully, luck intervened.

The only known artificial pandemic is thought to have started in 1977, ironically out of concern that a natural pandemic was imminent. That year a human H1N1 flu strain, dubbed the Russian flu because it was first identified there, reappeared almost simultaneously in Russia and China and circled the globe. Happily, it was very mild and bizarrely it only seriously affected people under the age of twenty-six. The only logical explanation was that anyone born before 1959, the last time the strain had been known to circulate, had built up some immunity to it. Indeed, when it was later genetically analysed, the 1977 strain was found to be practically identical to the 1959 H1N1 strain.[22]

Suspicious Western scientists questioned where this strain had been hiding between 1958 and 1976. Flu viruses mutate over about twenty years, so had this one been sitting in a Chinese or Russian deep freeze and then been used to develop a vaccine against the H1N1 flu? Had there been a lab accident? Was it possible that researchers and their families had become infected accidentally in the laboratory and allowed the virus to escape?

Epidemiologists must be medical detectives but in this case the politics of the age coloured their hypotheses. This was 1977. Jimmy Carter had just been inaugurated, the nuclear arms race was hot, terrorism and hijackings of planes were rife. The Soviet Union was known to be producing weapon-grade pathogens of anthrax, smallpox and other diseases and stories had been put around that agents were looking for the 1918 pandemic H1N1 flu strain in old ice houses where victims had been buried. The Western powers leapt to the conclusion that the pandemic was biowarfare.

What is certain, though, is that an H1N1 swine flu strain had emerged the previous year (1976), seriously infecting 230 American soldiers, hospitalising thirteen and killing one at the Fort Dix military camp in New Jersey. The spectre of the re-emergence of the deadly 1918 flu pandemic which killed millions of Americans triggered an unprecedented effort to immunise all Americans. There had also been major outbreaks first at a US air force base in England and then in one at a military camp in Colorado in 1977. All suggested biowarfare. It is now widely accepted that the pandemic had been caused by a vaccine trial in Russia or China that had gone wrong.[23]

Biowarfare researchers Michelle Rozo and Gifi Gronvall, working for the US government, reviewed the evidence in 2015 and all but dismissed the biowarfare theory, arguing that the unnatural origin of the evidence and its temperature sensitivity all suggested laboratory manipulation. But there was still a mystery: the fact that the pandemic broke out in China more or less at the same time as Russia suggested that this was not a single lab accident, and that it was linked to live virus vaccine trials which were taking place at the time.[24]

* * *

In late 2011 two teams of scientists supercharged the debate about pandemics starting accidentally. US virologist Yoshihiro Kawaoka and colleagues at the University of Wisconsin-Madison, and Ron Fouchier of Erasmus University in the Netherlands, separately showed how by manipulating just a few genes it was possible to make H5N1, a highly virulent bird flu virus which humans cannot normally contract, transmissible through the air between mammals.

Fouchier and Kawaoka were two of a new breed of virologists pushing the limits of knowledge and leading an intense, still active debate about how to prevent future pandemics. Their reasoning was that by engineering a deadlier flu virus they would enable science to better understand the constantly mutating nature of the pathogen and allow researchers to understand how pandemic viruses evolve. That way, they suggested, scientists would be able to make predictions about and prepare for future pandemics, and develop countermeasures to newly emerging ones. Mutating the flu virus was risky, they agreed, but given the risk of pandemics, doing nothing was even riskier.

They were backed by Anthony Fauci. With others he argued that creating potentially dangerous mutations in viruses was necessary to protect humanity. 'We cannot predict whether or not something will arise naturally, nor when or where it might appear. Given these uncertainties, important information and insights can come from generating a potentially dangerous virus in the laboratory,' they wrote in the *Washington Post*.[25]

The reaction from other scientists was swift and mostly critical. Life science 'gain-of-function' research like this is highly controversial, because as much as it may be intended for the benefit of humanity, it can equally be misapplied to do harm.[26] Making an airborne-transmittable version of H5N1 avian flu could be catastrophic for humanity if released.

Scientists were – and still are – split. Some supported Fouchier and Kawaoka, provided they did the research in strictly regulated and controlled conditions. Others, mostly infectious disease experts in what was called the Cambridge Working Group, were horrified.[27] This work, they said, was 'reckless' and of little benefit to society. The risks of an accidental, or even deliberate, release from a laboratory had, they said, the potential to kill many millions of people.[28] The US government sided with caution and in 2014 imposed a moratorium, but in 2017 the Trump administration lifted it.

In the decade since Fouchier and Kawaoka embarked on their 'gain of function' experiments, scientists working for unregulated, anonymous states, biotech and pharmaceutical companies, universities and others have been conducting similar secret experiments to observe how viruses, bacteria and other lethal pathogens like SARS and MERS, plague, anthrax, botulism, ricin, Ebola and Marburg may behave when they are enhanced and made more virulent or more transmissible. Within weeks of Mpox spreading around the world in 2022, virologists were trying to equip the relatively mild strain of the virus with a more lethal one. Other groups of scientists in London and Boston had applied to construct a lab-generated coronavirus with Omicron strains.

The argument for these 'gain-of-function' experiments is that the research may one day be needed to provide vaccines and to fight off the infectious diseases and prevent the pandemics of the future. But many scientists now question how valuable they are to science, and point out that they didn't prepare anyone for the Covid-19 pandemic. 'There are unimaginably many possible variants of a virus, of which researchers can identify only a few. Even if we stumble across one way a virus could mutate to become deadly, we might miss thousands of others,' MIT biologist and director of the Sculpting Evolution group Kevin Esvelt told *Vox* magazine in 2020.[29]

For some, like veteran US bio-campaigner Ronnie Cummins, these experiments are wide open to abuse. 'Unbeknownst to the public, a shadowy international network of virologists, gene engineers, military scientists and biotech entrepreneurs are weaponizing viruses and microorganisms in military and civilian labs under the euphemism of gain-of-function research … A growing arsenal of Frankenstein viruses and microorganisms have been created.'[30]

'Predicting how and when the next pandemic could arise is important, but tampering with viruses to do so is the wrong way to go about it,' says Princeton researcher and author Laura H. Kahn. 'There are other less risky ways of preventing pandemics than conducting gain-of-function research on pathogens. Many pathogens capable of causing human outbreaks originate in animals, and surveillance of wild and domestic animals for signs of illness makes sense.'[31]

* * *

One man who knows just how close the world has come to a catastrophic man-made pandemic is Colonel Kanatzhan Alibekov, for many years deputy director of Biopreparat, the old Soviet Union's massive biowarfare operation. Alibekov was in charge of weaponising vaccine-resistant versions of diseases like smallpox, HIV, plague, anthrax, Marburg and Ebola. Dubbed 'the ultimate killer' by the Western press, he defected to the US in 1992, anglicised his name to Ken Alibek, testified before the US Senate and revealed how at least seventeen countries were experimenting with pathogens which, should they escape, could lead to widespread disease. He was also in charge of what he describes as one of the 'most loathsome places on earth'. 'Rebirth island' in the chemically polluted and shrunken Aral Sea divides what is now Kazakhstan and Uzbekistan and is now deserted and nearly impossible to get to. But in 1982, when he was based there, it was a secret test centre for biological weapons.

Once in the US, he gave the CIA details of what is called the 'Sverdlovsk incident'. This started in an anonymous building on the southern edge of the city of that name, 160 kilometres east of Moscow. Here the Soviet Union was producing industrial quantities of anthrax for the military. In March 1979 a technician in the factory about to finish work for the night left a note for his supervisor saying a filter had been blocked. 'Replacement needed,' his note simply read.

But the note was not seen and when the machines were restarted a fine dust containing anthrax spores and chemical additives spewed over part of the town for several hours. Over the next few days many workers in a factory opposite the anthrax plant fell ill and died and hundreds more were violently sick. The story was put out that people had eaten anthrax-contaminated meat sold on the black market, but the truth that they had inhaled anthrax – a much more serious illness – was confirmed in 1992 by Boris Yeltsin, who had been the city's Communist Party leader at the time of the incident and had gone on to become the Soviet president.[32]

Alibek also revealed that early 'gain of function' research was underway on Rebirth Island to create entirely new life-forms. The goal, he wrote, was to insert genes from one virus into another to create an even more lethal virus. By the year before he defected, Soviet scientists were researching how to insert lethal Ebola and Marburg cells into smallpox virus. In 1989 he told how he came up with a list of biological weapons that would be used by the Soviet Union in future wars. 'We decided to replace brucellosis and Q fever with newer agents. Brucellosis would be replaced by glanders, a more efficient weapon. And instead of Q fever, I'm sorry to say, I suggested Marburg virus, a deadly hemorrhagic fever … Several other agents were under development, including Lassa fever, Ebola,

Machupo virus, Bolivian hemorrhagic fever, Argentine hemorrhagic fever, and Russian spring-summer encephalitis.'[33]

* * *

In the spring of 2012 three Chinese miners were asked to clear out metre-deep piles of bat guano from a network of old copper mines in Mojiang, Yunnan province. It would have been a foul job in a stinking, airless space and after two weeks of digging all three had picked up a severe pneumonia-like disease eerily similar to Covid-19. Three younger men took over and they too had breathing problems, coughs and fevers within a week. All six were admitted to Kunming Medical University, more than 150 kilometres away where they were put on ventilators. But three of them died within a few months, possibly becoming the first victims of the Covid-19 pandemic and the subjects of intense scrutiny by scientific investigators.

The Kunming doctors were baffled. The six had clearly been infected by inhaling dust from bat droppings. But when tested for diseases including Japanese encephalitis, Nipah and SARS – the coronavirus disease that had started in Hong Kong in 2003 and spread to eighteen countries – the results had all come back negative. Blood samples were sent for antibody testing to China's leading bat researcher, Professor Shi Zhengli, at the Wuhan virology institute, a world centre of coronavirus research and the only laboratory in China able to safely handle viruses like Ebola, bird flu and HIV. She concluded that it was an unknown 'SARS-like' virus derived from a horseshoe bat and it was given the name RaTG13, which referred to when and where it had been found.

The miners' illness was written up in great detail in a master's thesis by Li Xu of Kunming Medical University, one of the doctors who had treated them.[34] Separately, virus hunter scientists were sent by the Wuhan Institute to the mine to collect hundreds of samples of bat saliva and faeces. From these, nine coronaviruses were detected, of which one was RaTG13. But from then on little is certain. Information on the state of the samples they collected and the nature of any studies on them is conflicting, disputed and obscured by vested interests, and cloaked in medical and political mystery.

According to the WHO's official investigation, Professor Shi's colleagues went to the mineshaft seven times over the next three years to search for novel viruses for the US-funded PREDICT programme.[35] None, they told the WHO, were the genetic progenitor virus of SARS-CoV-2, but one was a SARS-like virus, 96.2 per cent the same, which was not related to Covid-19 but was by far the closest genetic relative yet found to it.

Could this have been the source of Covid-19? The Mojiang Miners' Passage hypothesis, first proposed by virologist Jonathan Latham and geneticist Allison Wilson, suggests that the virus could have emerged more or less naturally and then been worked on in the Wuhan labs before somehow escaping. It is just one of many serious explanations offered for the arrival of SARS-Cov-2, the strain of coronavirus that causes Covid-19.

Covid-19's origin has become the ultimate scientific whodunnit, dividing scientists, politicians and governments, and giving rise to conspiracy theories and accusations of cover-ups and personal attacks. But as Australian virologist Kennedy Shortridge found when investigating avian flu outbreaks in Hong Kong in the 1980s, if you want to determine the origin of a disease it is just as important to understand the social and political context of the time it emerged as the genetic makeup of the virus itself. Here, the big picture on the eve of Covid-19 being found in the Wuhan wet market in December 2019 was that China was seeking to match and overtake the US and Europe in medical and food technologies, genetic engineering, bio-weaponry and life sciences.

Its only Level-4 laboratory had just been built in Wuhan, and accreditation to research the world's most dangerous pathogens, like Ebola, Nipah and Marburg, had only been granted in 2018. It had brilliant researchers, but few of them had much experience working in high-level labs and most were under pressure to perform cutting-edge research.

Meanwhile, southern China's massive urban consumer society was adopting meat-based diets and demanding not just cheap poultry and pork, but exotic animals like civets, porcupines, pangolins, raccoon dogs, snakes and bamboo rats, which were mostly bred for food and medicine in thousands of small but intensively run wildlife farms. Traders, too, were smuggling in captive-bred and forest-caught wild animals from neighbouring Laos, Vietnam, Cambodia and even Africa.

In this time of great social, environmental and scientific upheaval the conditions were perfect for a new virus to emerge from a market, farm or laboratory. Even as China's scientists were pushing research boundaries, its farmers were intensifying animal breeding and the rearing of wild animals in unnatural conditions, and traders were coming into closer contact with animals carrying unknown viruses.

But three years' of investigations by governments, ecologists, journalists and global institutions have found no smoking gun. Thousands of animals from hundreds of species have been tested for the virus, but it has still not been found. We still do not know definitively how, where or even when Covid-19 originated.

Nevertheless, the idea that it was engineered and then escaped from the Wuhan laboratory is powerful and has caught the Western imagination. The Wuhan lab, after all, was the only one in Asia known to have been working with novel Sars-like viruses, and specifically working to enhance them. The fact that China will not open its databases is damning, as is the fact that its leading coronavirus researchers, some partly funded with US money, were splicing together strains to discover how they might become more infectious to humans.

Was there a cover-up? Yes. Have there been mishaps and accidents in the Wuhan labs? Yes. Could a virus like RaTG13 found in the Mojiang cave have been manipulated? Yes. Was the lab conducting risky experiments? Yes. Could the genome have been synthesised seamlessly without leaving a trace? Yes.

But all of that is circumstantial evidence. The reality is that we may never know for certain. As of early 2023 all scientific research into Covid-19's origins has stalled. There is no technology that can accurately distinguish between an engineered sequence and a natural genome sequence. There are just too many ways to manipulate a genome without leaving a signature.

Until the technology arrives, or courts force access to so-far closed databases, or a whistleblower produces absolute proof, the most likely origin remains the natural zoonotic spillover of a virus from an animal to a human. Virology labs are dangerous and Covid-19 could certainly have leaked from the one at Wuhan, but after so much investigation we must trust the knowledge of the world's leading virologists, who remain broadly certain it was a natural event – albeit one almost certainly aided by human action.

Hard questions must be asked of the way gain-of-function experiments are devised and conducted, and labs must be reined in, but experience suggests that nature is more likely to come up with a surprise than humans are.

But nearly forty years after Janet Parker died a gruesome death in Birmingham following a laboratory escape of the smallpox virus, the age of lab escapes is far from over. In 2016 Canadian scientists funded by an American biotech company went on the web and bought the fragments of DNA necessary to make a closely related but extinct virus known as horsepox.[36] Using 'synthetic biology' techniques, they proceeded to show how a small team of biologists 'without exceptional knowledge or skills, significant funds or significant time' could recreate the smallpox virus for less than $100,000. The era of DIY pathogens had started.[37]

In theory, only a very small stock of smallpox virus is held in two ultra-secure labs, one in the US, another in Russia. It is kept, it is said, just in case the disease were ever to return and a vaccine were needed. In reality, many countries almost certainly hold some. The point about safety was well made in November 2021, when several vials labelled 'smallpox' were found by a worker cleaning out an old freezer in a vaccine lab in Pennsylvania.[38]

How many more forgotten pathogens could there be waiting to be found in the world's many laboratories? Predicting disaster is hard, but as we shall see, it's getting easier.

PREPARE TO PREVENT

The river Cavu on the French Mediterranean island of Corsica descends from granite mountains through dense pine and oak forests in a series of waterfalls, rapids and quiet stretches. It is famous for its pools of crystal-clear turquoise water. Locals swim in them, few walkers can resist plunging in, and nowadays tourists flock to the Cavu's banks to enjoy the dragonflies and pondlife insects that skim over the water.

But in 2013 and again in 2015 hundreds of locals and tourists who had swum in the Cavu contracted schistosomiasis, a debilitating disease also known as bilharzia, which causes chills and anaemia as well as liver and bladder damage. It affects more than 200 million people, mainly in tropical Africa and Asia, every year and is caused by a worm released by snails.

How did schistosomiasis, classed by the WHO as an 'emerging zoonotic disease', contaminate the pristine waters of the Cavu? No one thought that a snail-borne tropical disease like this would appear in Europe, let alone make itself at home in a French mountain river. Corsica had always been considered well outside the geographic range of schistosomiasis because of the near-freezing temperatures of its rivers in the winter.

Discovering how it got there and then working out how to stop it proved hard. French doctors had seen nothing like this before and were not trained to diagnose or treat the disease, local ecologists and parasite experts were baffled, and vets were surprised. But a team of specialists was brought together and the facts of the mystery were established: first, local freshwater snails had somehow become the host for the tiny larvae of the parasitical schistosoma flatworm;[1] second, none of the affected people had been recently to tropical or subtropical countries; third, they were linked only by swimming in the river. The disease had only ever been seen in Corsica in cattle, and then very rarely.

But the explanation they eventually arrived at suggested that it had taken human, animal and environmental factors for it to emerge there and then. The larvae of the parasitical worm were probably brought to Corsica by a tourist who had been infected while swimming in Senegal, and a series of warm winters and heavier-than-usual rainfall in Corsica had likely raised water temperatures and increased the abundance of the host snail and its parasite worms. In short, the disease had broken out when a complex mix of human, animal, local, planetary and environmental forces had combined.[2]

Mysterious diseases are increasingly turning up in new places. Climate change, the cutting down of forests and suburban housing encroaching on wild lands are together thought to have encouraged Lyme disease to establish itself in Michigan. Doctors and environmentalists worked together there to see how a shifting ecology was making it possible for a disease to cross into a human population.

Human health, it is now better understood, is intimately connected to the health of animals and the environment. As humans modify earth's natural systems – the air, water, biodiversity and climate – so the geography of diseases like malaria, Lyme disease, West Nile virus, Zika, yellow fever, SARS, Nipah and Hendra is also changing. In 2022 researchers showed how the deadly Hendra virus, which attacks horses and humans, could be accurately predicted two years in advance. They found that bats shed more of the virus depending on drought, habitat loss and the availability of food.

'The harms we inflict on our planetary systems now threaten our very existence as a species,' says Richard Horton, editor-in-chief of the *Lancet* family of medical journals, who coined the term 'planetary health' in March 2014 and calls for a holistic approach to health. 'Our patterns of overconsumption are unsustainable and will ultimately cause the collapse of our civilisation. The gains made in health and well-being over recent centuries, including through public health actions, are not irreversible; they can easily be lost, a lesson we have failed to learn from previous civilisations.'[3]

Planetary health – or, as it is sometimes called, one health – is an emerging approach to understanding the way we interact with nature. As it stands, the health of people, animals and the planet are treated separately. Doctors look after human diseases, vets exclusively take care of animal health and the natural world is left mostly to conservationists and politicians. But the interdependence of the three is rarely considered.

What is needed to avoid another SARS or Covid-19, bird flu or Ebola, say Horton and others, is a fusion of veterinary, human and environmental knowledge. Pandemic prevention needs surveillance and collaboration, data sharing and new thinking. You can't look at diseases of humans in isolation from diseases of wildlife, any more than you can look at diseases of wildlife in isolation from changes in the environment. Epidemics, whether of people or animals, don't just happen, says Horton. 'They are increasingly a result of things that people do to nature. If you can prevent the disease in the animal, and if you can prevent the disease in the environment, it will never get to the person.'[4]

A radical approach to tackling health is needed because never before have so many people depended on so many animals for so much food; nor has the environment ever been so stretched to provide for both people and wild animals. With human populations reaching 8 billion in 2022, and around 33 billion domesticated cattle, pigs, sheep and poultry, and the global environment struggling, the health of plants, animals and humans must be seen as one.

Ways to pre-empt and handle pandemics have changed little in 1,000 years. Pandemics are still treated as inherently unpredictable, and involve identifying, quarantining and isolating infected people and, hopefully, vaccinating others. Animal and plant pandemics are handled brutally – by killing infected animals and using chemical pesticides.[5] A radical new approach to ensuring global health is needed because never before have so many people depended on so many animals, or has the environment been so stretched to produce food. Demand for animal proteins is surging, and, as a result, new infectious diseases which originate in both farmed and wild animals are emerging. Instead of seeing zoonotic diseases, antimicrobial resistance,[6] foodborne illnesses, food insecurity and climate change as separate problems, we should understand that are all connected.

Princeton researcher Laura Kahn reminds us that divisions between physicians and veterinarians have only opened recently. It was the great German physician and Victorian pathologist Rudolf Virchow, she says, 'who in 1858 coined the term "zoonosis", and said, ' "between animal and human medicine there are no dividing lines – nor should there be." '[7]

Animals, it is now recognised, act as sentinels for environmental contamination, but the signs they highlight are typically overlooked. Pets share people's homes and are vulnerable to similar environmental contaminants but instead of the 'whack-a-mole' approach now employed where countries wait for diseases to arrive and then react to them, what if they were understood to be entirely predictable, the places that they were most likely to strike were known in advance and people were taught to watch out and prepare for diseases? What, indeed, if we understood both viruses and ecology better and the relationship between nature and disease?

It is far from impossible. In the last twenty years, the power of computers, AI, machine learning and increased knowledge about ecology, viruses and other species has made it much more possible to predict where most of the best-known dangerous pathogens are likely to strike and be ready for them with vaccines and drugs.

* * *

If stopping future pandemics is not possible, being prepared for them may be the best we can do. That means surveillance must be extended to people who work in forests, on farms handling animals and in virology laboratories – anywhere people might come into close contact with pathogens. Researchers can now detect viruses in waste water or air.

One man who has had as much experience as anyone in trying to prepare for pandemics and head them off before they start is Dennis Carroll, who for years led the US government's attempts to anticipate avian flu and other dangerous diseases like Ebola and HIV/Aids. Now in his seventies, he has been called the 'godfather of infectious disease' and 'king of the virus hunters', but with his shoulder-length white hair he cuts the image of an Old Testament prophet.

Carroll ran what was, until it was closed down by President Trump in 2019, the forerunner of a global early warning system for new viruses. The $200 million Predict programme sent scores of researchers from universities, local communities, conservation groups and natural history museums around the world deep into the caves and forests of the Amazon, Congo Basin and Southeast Asia with orders to collect mucus, urine and saliva samples from thousands of bird and mammal species thought most likely to be reservoirs of disease. Together they identified more than 1,200 new viruses, including more than 160 novel coronaviruses.

'Viruses are even more diverse than mammals,' he told me in some awe at their complexity and abundance, but also in astonishment at how little we know about them. 'More than 260 are so far known in humans but they are some of the oldest forms of life on Earth and together comprise 60 per cent of the Earth's living matter. We think at least 1.5 million live in mammals and birds. The unknown ones represent 99.9 per cent of potential zoonoses and usually remain undetected until they cause disease in humans.'[8]

Most are quite harmless to humans but our ignorance is dangerous, because our destruction of the natural world makes it more likely that new ones will emerge and spill over into human populations, he says. 'Every time we look for viruses we find new things, and they often challenge our understanding.'[9]

Carroll now chairs the Global Virome project, an ambitious $4 billion plan to build on Predict and discover and genetically record all the world's million or more unknown viruses that might threaten humanity. He thinks of it as an 'atlas of viruses' and 'the beginning of the end of the pandemic era'. Its aim, he says, is to prepare proactively for viruses to strike.

Scouring the world's species for unknown pathogens would be a mammoth enterprise, even more ambitious than the Human Genome project, which took thirteen years to map all the genes of the human genome. Nevertheless, it is feasible and, when the costs of Covid-19 and the disruption it has caused are added up, it makes sense to many economists.

'We need to understand viruses and their ecosystems better, and gain a better understanding of hotspots. Compare weather forecasting: fifty years ago it was very limited, we could forecast a hurricane two days out. Now we can forecast them on an annual basis, pick them up off the coast of West Africa, and make pretty precise predictions. Disease prediction has so far relied on surveillance and preparedness. Surveillance has primarily focused on identifying early cases of a virus, identifying the index – or first – case and then responding. But any virus that poses a future threat already exists. So why wait for it?' says Carroll.[10]

Carroll makes a compelling case. 'We need to move beyond the era of medicate-vaccinate-eradicate and shine a spotlight on the wider "parascape". Rather than focus on the known major pathogens, we should embark on the mammoth task of documenting all parasites, focusing on unknown infections, particularly those in reservoir hosts.'[11]

'We have some data but we need much more and we need to run it through models like meteorologists do. We want to move the world of virology from being a Mom-and-Pop operation. There are 4,500 coronaviruses alone. Why can't we document them in their entirety? Predict showed us we could do it.'[12]

It would be a vastly expensive exercise generating almost unimaginable quantities of data, but the prize, he says, would be an open-access atlas of the genetic make-up of all the world's most dangerous viruses, which would help us to better prepare for disease outbreaks and enable drug companies to develop broad-spectrum vaccines and drugs in advance.

With millions of records, scientists might be able to pinpoint when parasites reach higher latitudes, viruses cross species barriers for the first time, or warmer temperatures spark fungal epidemics, on timescales of just weeks to months. At long last, outbreak or pandemic forecasting might be nearly as accurate as a ten-day weather forecast.

Above all, Carroll says, we should anticipate humans having a hand in the emergence of any new infectious disease. Working with bird flu in Southeast Asia convinced him that people becoming wealthier and eating more meat in China was behind many disease outbreaks. 'Avian flu was a direct consequence of how much poultry was being produced to feed people. If you look at China today it produces something in the order of 15–20 billion poultry a year, but if you went back to the 1960s you see at best only a few hundred million were under production.'[13]

A spillover event, he says, is not a consequence of the virus itself, but of the way humans behave.

> Viruses do not spread by themselves; we enable them to
> spill over and spread by the way we interact with ecosystems
> around us. The one thing we know with certainty is that our
> interaction with wildlife and the eco systems are increasingly
> becoming more dynamic and impactful. As we move further
> into the twenty-first century, and our population increases from
> 8 to 12 billion people, this combination of biologic risk and
> behaviour risk is going to result in intensification of spillovers
> with new novel viruses causing epidemics and pandemics with
> greater frequency then we have ever seen in human history
> before.

He sums up the human dilemma:

> Pandemics are not God-ordained events, they are as a direct
> consequence of the way we live. They are preventable, and if we
> pay closer attention to the way we live, we can be much more
> effective at minimising the opportunities for these spillover
> events to happen.[14]

* * *

Predicting and preventing pandemics has, since Covid-19, become a global priority But data on its own is useless, says US immunologist Rick Bright, working with the WHO. 'The data is siloed, Balkanised and fragmented. We have amazing genomic surveillance and epidemiological data. We also have data from academia and the private sector. There's gold mines and oil fields of data but it's absolutely useless on its own.'[15]

Rather than spend billions of dollars compiling a global database of viruses that are by nature constantly evolving and may or may not enable vaccines and treatments to be developed, would it not be better to study where diseases are most likely to emerge? I went back to Thomas Gillespie, who had been working for much of the pandemic in equatorial Africa. We had last spoken at the start of the Covid pandemic. 'Diseases don't emerge from just anywhere. Often they come from rainforest edges and places of great diversity, where humans and animal species intersect and there is a great diversity of species like bats and rats which are known to transmit diseases. [They] are more likely to spill over from animals to humans, in known hotspot places which are closely linked to environmental change such as deforestation. Tropical rainforests are exceptionally important in this regard.'[16]

'Logging and subsistence agriculture in Africa for instance are reducing habitat for wild primates leaving them less forest to forage in. That can make them unhealthy and more susceptible to disease. And it may drive them to risk encounters with humans, raising risks of the exchange of pathogens.'

He speculated that Covid-19 could even have emerged after large-scale land change in China. 'Everyone has been talking about the problem of the wet market in Wuhan, but what about the nearby Three Gorges dam, the world's largest hydroelectric power station, built on the Yangtze River in an area that was previously secondary forest and farmland? Many of the animals that used to live in that area likely died when their habitat was destroyed, but bats can fly. Where did they go? How did they adapt?'[17]

Our knowledge of disease hotspots like the edge of forests, or certain parts of China, Africa and Latin America that are being rapidly transformed, is improving thanks to painstaking field research and better surveillance. It has enabled researchers like Gillespie and Rick Ostfeld, mentioned in Chapter 15, to narrow down the geography of diseases. But it gets more complicated because it means taking into account the social and environmental changes happening in the places they are most likely to emerge, and seeing what animals are known or likely to be found in any one location.

Just how complicated, but also how rewarding, it can be to predict a disease outbreak can be seen with Ebola. Anticipating it is particularly important because it is one of the most lethal diseases in the world and because it has started to emerge in densely populated cities after years of being confined to small populations in forested West and Central Africa. Since it first emerged in the 1970s, it has broken out forty-odd times in seven countries, often thousands of kilometres apart. Then it has disappeared, sometimes for years, baffling governments and disease experts, who can only try to respond as fast as possible. Now the outbreaks appear to be bigger and more frequent.

Given good diverse data, this notoriously random zoonotic disease, which is passed to humans via primates and probably bats, may actually be quite predictable, says David Redding, a researcher at the ZSL Institute of Zoology in London.[18] He and colleagues at Lancaster University have built a computer model which factors in a huge range of data, including information about the animals that carry Ebola, the speed of technological and social change like urban expansion, as well as the expected changes to climate, the temperature, rainfall, types of habitat, even the transport links between places.

Redding has accurately predicted where the last three outbreaks would emerge, though not their precise timing, by seeing how changes to ecosystems and human societies combine. His maps show Ebola hotspots in the expected equatorial places like Gabon and the Democratic Republic of Congo, but also in countries that have never had outbreaks before like Nigeria and Ghana. By including climate change data, it is also possible to predict how Ebola will shift its range.

'It's too early to say whether we have captured the true pattern of risk. We have used our understanding of how climate and habitat create the conditions suitable for the host animal species which carry the Ebola virus to exist and then where people and these animals are likely to contact each other.'[19]

'There is no reason why this model should not be used to predict outbreaks of more than two hundred other known zoonotic diseases,' says Kate Jones, chair of ecology and biodiversity at UCL, who worked with Redding.[20]

Tracking some individual diseases already takes place. Seasonal flu viruses, which are continuously changing, are followed remarkably successfully by governments and flu centres as they travel around the world every year.[21] The data enables drug companies and governments to prepare hundreds of millions of doses to be manufactured ahead of flu seasons.

But wider checks on changes taking place in ecosystems and animal diseases are also needed as zoonotic diseases increase and the threat of future pandemics grows. Conservation groups want records kept of animals sold in wildlife markets, while others envisage laboratories and public and private institutions sharing data in a global early pandemic warning system.

* * *

With so many people in the world having little or no access to basic healthcare and dying of undetected causes, are not massive high-tech data crunching, machine learning, genomic testing and all the other ambitious proposals to ramp up surveillance for potential pandemic pathogens not missing the point? For many in developing countries at least, by far the most cost-effective and efficient way to prepare for pandemics and stop diseases spreading is to address poverty and public health. Investment in hospitals and providing communities with clean water and sanitation would immediately improve tens of millions of lives and stop many diseases in their tracks for a paltry $10 billion a year, says the WHO – a snip compared to the trillions that the Covid pandemic has cost.[22]

The situation was well put at the height of the Covid pandemic by Helen Clark, former prime minister of New Zealand and co-chair of the Independent Panel for Pandemic Preparedness and Response. 'To provide every person in the world with access to clean water and safe sanitation wouldn't break the bank. It has to be prioritised. Water and sanitation are right up there as among the basics for a decent life.'[23]

Keeping solutions simple is vital, say experienced future pandemic spotters. Nothing protects people more than vigilance, says Jonathan Quick, author of *The End of Pandemics* and director of Pandemic Preparedness and Prevention at the Rockefeller Foundation. He tells me: 'We can have all the medications and knowledge available to heal the sick, but if we don't build strong health systems we will continue to see [pandemics] … which cause needless suffering and death. We can enable people and countries to thrive, or continue to lurch from one public health crisis to another instead of stopping them all.'[24]

Quick is old-school. 'The single most important thing is actually the most low-tech. We have to get [the] front line of healthcare all over the world listened to by the next level up. With Covid-19, the next level up was in denial. To avoid pandemics, it needs vigilance all the way up and then rapid action. You have to be on the ground. What is needed is to set up a very solid and strong surveillance system that enables people to detect these pathogens in real time, and then make this information available.'[25]

There is consensus that a safer world requires a better global early-warning system, using genomic surveillance, to spot the spread of pathogens and track new variants and viruses as they evolve. But it's not enough to throw money at vaccines, or digital tools, without addressing the causes of pandemics. Says Aaron Bernstein, leader of the Harvard T. H. Chan School of Public Health: 'We must invest in preventing pandemics before they begin. Actions that target the root causes will protect our health, stabilise the climate and come at a fraction of the cost of what it has taken to respond to Covid-19.'[26]

'The cost of public health preparedness is a tiny fraction of the price of disaster,' says Tom Frieden, former director of the CDC: 'Pandemics aren't inevitable. We can prevent another [one]. But unless the underlying causes are addressed, the same mistakes will continue to be made and history will repeat itself. Infectious diseases tend to be guided missiles aimed at the poor and disenfranchised. True to form, Covid has been a pandemic of inequality, injustice, and inequity.'[27]

Nearly two years into a coronavirus pandemic that has killed more than 5 million people and plunged 100 million people into deepest poverty, every country remains dangerously unprepared to respond to future pandemic threats, concludes Tom Frieden. 'We face a common enemy – dangerous microbes. They don't wait, and coronavirus isn't the only one out there.'[28]

THE HEALTHY HUMAN

I am practising shinrin-yoku, or 'forest bathing', in some woodland near where I live. A therapist who normally conducts sessions in Central Park, New York, has told me online to leave behind my phone, camera and other distractions and talk to no one. I should wander, breathe deeply, listen to the wind, admire the dappled light, feel the moss, sniff the sweet, rich earth and listen to the birds and wildlife as I immerse myself in this treescape. It is to be a pleasant, gentle, mindful meditation aimed to still the mind and stimulate the senses.

'Don't think about it. Inhale it. Just be with the trees,' were her last commands.

Despite the dangers of tripping over roots, being bitten by ants and getting muddy (this is Wales!), forest bathing like this has become a worldwide phenomenon, relaxing frazzled urban minds and bodies overwhelmed by technology and the rush of life. I've walked through this wood hundreds of times over the years, but just stopping, sitting and watching the little Morlas brook, examining a leaf or deliberately smelling the rich earth, does indeed seem to clear the head, improve the mood and soothe the body. It is a visual and olfactory treat, a psychological and physical tonic for the coming day.

The Covid-19 pandemic helped us understand how the human disturbance of nature and the intensive farming of animals can lead to diseases jumping from species to species. But busy lives and lifestyles – people in high-income countries spend up to 90 per cent of their time indoors – makes it easy to forget that both planetary and individual health depends entirely on the natural environment. Now we are learning, too, about the central roles that the environment and lifestyle play in health and human well-being.

All cultures recognise an instinctive connection between nature and health but in the past forty years an avalanche of studies – some better than others – have provided the evidence that ought to persuade governments and the medical profession to take note and act. Therapies which encourage people to expose themselves to the natural environment might once have been widely dismissed as esoteric and having spiritual overtones, but mainstream healthcare is now beginning to take notice of evidence that nature heals.

Today, led by psychiatrists, there are a bewildering number of 'eco-therapies' intended to 'reconnect' people with their 'inner' and 'outer' natures and help people overcome stress and mental disorders. Anxious or depressed people are asked to 'slow walk', embrace trees, meditate, view the night sky and watch clouds.

The medical profession has come late to the party but gardening and fresh air are now being prescribed to help some people with dementia and mental health struggles; troubled teenagers with behaviour problems are successfully sent on wilderness programmes; there are apps to help people benefit from sitting by the sea and waterfalls; 'green care' – hospital treatment programmes that take place in natural surroundings – is used to help people recover from strokes as well as to help patients with autism, learning disabilities and dementia. Playing with animals, planting trees, even growing tomatoes have all been found to create a sense of optimism and the future, while digging releases stressed workers and stargazing creates a positive mood.

Heading to the forest for a bath certainly helped people cope with the pandemic. Amanda Heywood, a young American teacher who has lived in Tokyo for five years, told me how it saved her sanity when she came out of months of Covid-19 quarantine with low energy and mixed-up emotions. Like many others, she said she felt burned out with stress, lonely and purposeless. Going with others once a week to the Mount Takao forest trails just outside Tokyo gave her the space to recover from the trauma of the pandemic and become able to face life in the largest conurbation in the world.

Nor does forest healing always need professional therapists. National forestry companies in Germany,[1] Ireland,[2] the UK and Italy have all reported great increases in the number of people who took to the trees and went hiking in a time of social isolation. In what may prove one of the most positive post-Covid changes,[3] people have learned to appreciate nature. US researchers have reported an 'unprecedented' increase in the number of people spending time in forests and countryside.[4] Similarly, European countries report enormous new interest in gardening, 'rewilding', growing houseplants, walking and outdoor yoga. It is as if we are hard-wired to turn to nature, the evolutionary home of *Homo sapiens*, for mental and physical reassurance and strength in difficult times.

Japan, which has one of the highest suicide rates of any high-income country, has led the world in the modern scientific study of nature's recuperative powers. The government, aware of the country's crowded cities and work stress, has since the early 1980s ploughed money into medical research into the health and well-being benefits of forests in particular.

Miyazaki Yoshifum, a professor at Chiba University's Centre for Environment, Health and Field Sciences, claims to have coined the term 'forest bathing' in 2003. He and other researchers from the Hokkaido University School of Medicine reportedly travelled in the late 1980s to Yaku island, a lush-green, semi-tropical island off the southern tip of Japan famous for its ancient cedar and cypress trees and its many thousands of plant species.[5] There they set about conducting experiments with diabetes sufferers, people with heart conditions, high-school students and the lonely and depressed.

Much more research is needed, says Miyazaki, but there is little doubt that spending time among trees or in the open air not only decreases blood glucose levels in diabetic patients, boosts immune systems, accelerates recovery from illness, increases energy and improves sleep, but also reduces heart and depressive symptoms and increases feelings of well-being. Miyazaki and others are careful not to say nature will cure anything and everything, only that it can restore people psychologically and emotionally as well as provide them with the immune system resilience to ward off some diseases.

Filtering out all the many physical and psychological factors that can determine feelings of well-being and health makes it hard to pinpoint whether it is the forest, the view, the air or the physical exercise – or all of them – which makes people feel better. Few studies have looked at the effects of exposure to nature over any length of time and the long-term effects claimed are often speculative. But in the short term, at least, by taking blood tests before and after experiences in nature, imaging the brain and analysing hormones, researchers have shown that there is barely any condition that contact with nature cannot improve.

Some studies appear to show conclusively that walks in the countryside improve mental disorders and ease respiratory diseases, migraines and depressions. The growing consensus is that exposure to green space in urban areas results in short-term psychological and physiological benefits – even though there is no agreement on how they work. One 2008 survey of the medical records of nearly 350,000 people in ninety-six Dutch doctors' surgeries showed that the prevalence of fifteen common illnesses depended on the closeness of green space within a kilometre of the patients' homes,[6] and that a stroll in the woods has been found to lower cortisol levels, pulse rate and blood pressure more than a walk through pleasant urban areas.

Studies showing nature's ability to help recuperation are now accumulating fast. A child's concentration appears to improve when they are in the open air. Andrea Faber Taylor and Frances Kuo at the University of Illinois at Urbana-Champaign, for example, found that children with attention-deficit hyperactivity disorder (ADHD) concentrated better after a walk in the park – about as well as if they had taken standard medication.[7] Walking through quiet and pleasant areas of town with less greenery did not work nearly so well.

But how does nature do it? Research suggests that the air in forests and wild places is particularly rich in volatile and other components normally absent in urban, built environments and that when we walk among trees we inhale natural antimicrobial and insecticidal chemicals known as phytocenes, which are given off by trees and plants to protect themselves against bugs, bacteria and diseases and which boost immune systems.[8]

Other studies point to the astonishing biodiversity of microorganisms present in the rural, as opposed to the urban air. Studies from the US and EU reckon there could be almost as many organisms in the air as are found in soils, with hundreds of thousands, even millions of bacteria and other microbes in every cubic metre of air above shrubs, and even more above places where animals are kept. Indian researchers have suggested that in forests there are phenomenal numbers of beneficial pollen grains, fungal spores, bacteria, mycelium, cysts, algal filaments and spores, and lichens.[9]

US author and biologist Joan Maloof, who directs the Old Growth forest network, refers to a study of air in the Sierra Nevada mountains in Northern California which showed that of the 120 chemical compounds found in the mountain forest air only seventy were identifiable. 'We are literally breathing things we don't understand,' she wrote in 2005. 'And when we lose our forests, we don't know what we are losing.'[10]

Belgian biologist Raf Aerts, meanwhile, has documented some of the recent studies showing that the exposure of infants to nature is linked to later reduced respiratory, heart and cancer mortality as well as the risk of developing schizophrenia. One study has shown how the greenness of a mother's neighbourhood in the months leading to birth may have a positive effect on the birth weight of their infants, and that living in a green part of a city has a positive effect on blood pressure in adolescents.[11]

Miyazaki, too, takes the long view: 'We need the forest now more than ever for our health. Although human beings and their direct ancestors have existed for approximately seven million years, we have spent over 99.99 per cent of that time living in nature. Our genes are adapted to nature, and they have not changed over the two or three centuries since the industrial revolution. Because we have bodies that are adapted to nature, living in modern society places us in a condition of stress,' he suggests.[12] '[Today] young people have less contact with nature than before, and it seems that they are more stressed than ever. Since our bodies are adapted to nature from the start, this result is unsurprising. Right now, depression among children is increasing,' he suggests.[13]

Graham Rook, professor of medical microbiology at University College London, has been key to helping us understand how the extraordinary diversity of microbes influences human health. In 2003 he debunked the compelling 'hygiene' theory, which since 1989 had suggested that the reason for soaring rates of multiple sclerosis, Crohn's disease, type 1 diabetes and asthma, as well as declines in the incidence of mumps, measles, TB and other infectious diseases, was that vaccines, antibiotics and improved hygiene were causing immune systems to malfunction in some way.

Rook came up with the delightfully named 'old friends' hypothesis. This proposed that modern life has compromised our hugely complex microbiome and that our immune systems may now incorrectly categorise harmless substances as a threat. He suggests that the organisms vital to the development of our immune and gut systems are the very ones that we were in contact with during early hunter-gatherer times more than 10,000 years ago, when our immune systems were developing. These billions of viruses, bacteria and helminths, which are naturally present in soil, water and food, also colonise the skin, gut and respiratory tracts of animals and humans. Early exposure to these 'friendly' microbes, proposes Rook, is necessary to train the human immune system to identify and react to allergens and threats.

But Rook goes further, arguing that humans depend on the microbes that they co-evolved with. Normally, beneficial ancient species of microorganisms would be acquired in the natural environment or passed down from mother to child, but humanity's abrupt move to cities and indoor environments and its growing isolation from the natural environment and use of antibiotics may together be changing us on a microbial level, he suggests. The crucial thing for health is contact with green space and the natural environment, and avoidance of antibiotics and things that limit that transmission of maternal microbiota to the infant.

It makes instinctive sense. We evolved in the natural environment and lived in shelters constructed from components of that environment. Until quite recently our homes were built with timber and thatch and rendered with mud and animal dung. The modern house, built with biocide-treated timber, plasterboard and plastic, has an alien microbiota that can, if the house is damp, include organisms that are toxic to us because they were not part of our evolutionary history. Gardening and walks in nature expose us to the microbiota that our physiology evolved to anticipate.'

He writes: 'Perhaps the major problem right now is the disruption of natural ecosystems by agriculture (especially monoculture), urbanisation, agricultural and industrial chemicals, and man-made climate change. All these factors are changing the microorganisms to which we are exposed, and by which we are colonised. We do not know how far these exposures can deviate safely from the exposures of our evolutionary past, on which we are in a state of evolved dependence.'

* * *

Bit by bit, study by study, the importance of the natural environment to human health and well-being is being refined, extended and better understood. In Denmark, people living more than one kilometre from a natural green environment were found to be more likely to be obese and less likely to exercise rigorously than those living within 300 metres. Another study found that doctors in urban areas with more trees on the street tended to prescribe fewer antidepressants than those in urban areas without trees. Older people are more likely to live longer if they live near walkable greenery-filled public areas, found one study. Quite simply, people are happier and have lower mental distress when they live closer to nature.

Many of these studies are too small to be reliable, but larger, more rigorous ones suggest much the same. Researchers at the Institute for European Environmental Policy reviewed 200 studies for Friends of the Earth Europe and reached the conclusion that being physically close to nature improves your health, even when controlling for other factors. They found that middle-aged men living in deprived urban areas with high amounts of green space had a much lower risk than similar groups living in equally deprived areas with less greenery.[14]

One bit of the health puzzle was put in place in 2020 when Finnish and Czech researchers got permission to replace the concrete and asphalt play areas in several inner-city Helsinki infant schools with hundreds of cubic metres of turf, soil and plants dug up from forest areas. The children were then encouraged to play in their newly forested school playgrounds for several hours a day and had their immune systems tested before and after their environment was changed. The results were striking.[15] It was a smallish study with just seventy-five children but within a month their immune systems were found to have greatly improved, with a big increase in the number and concentration of healthy microbes on the skin biome – the body's largest organ – and positive changes, too, in proteins and cells.

It convinced lead researcher Marja Roslund, from the University of Helsinki, that schools should rethink their environments. 'It is completely incomprehensible that nowadays our children play in yards consisting mostly of asphalt, sand, and plastic carpet. We should take care of our children and modify the living environment so that every child has the opportunity to play in biodiverse environments to protect the natural development of their immune system,' she said.[16]

The 'old friends' theory is now evolving into what other researchers are calling the 'biodiversity hypothesis', which suggests that contact with natural environments enriches the human microbiome, promotes immune balance and protects from allergy and inflammatory disorders. A global loss of biodiversity may be to blame for the dysfunctioning of the human immune system, resulting in allergic and inflammatory diseases around the world.

Some clues, again from Scandinavia, came from a ten-year study of genetically homogenous children on either side of the

Russia–Finland border. In the Second World War a large area of the region known as Karelia was transferred to Russia. Fifty years later, people on the Soviet side had carried on their rural, traditional lifestyle while those on the Finnish side of the border had modernised, with populations growing and urbanising, and people changing diets, living more sedentary lives and going out of doors far less.

The study found those on the Finnish side suffered appreciably more asthma, hay fever from birch pollen and skin diseases[17] – diseases that were almost non-existent on the Russian side. It was strong proof that the lack of exposure to natural environments was driving the allergy pandemic that was being experienced throughout the world.

Of course, there are many factors in play when it comes to health, but the overriding conclusion is that the alarming rise in obesity, sedentary lifestyles and mental ill health across the developed world has resulted in an urgent desire to understand how the environment affects us.

* * *

But what's new? From the Hanging Gardens of Babylon in Neolithic Iraq 8,000 years ago and modern-day Buddhist gardens in Japan, through to the 'father of modern medicine' Hippocrates and Pliny the Younger in ancient Greece, the sacred groves of India and the garden city movements, access to nature has been always been known and respected as a fundamental human need, the provider of health and well-being. Somewhere in the twentieth century wealthy countries seemed to forget that it was necessary either physically or psychologically, with catastrophic results for health.

We now see a widening gap between people and the natural environment. Cities are generally bigger and denser today, with more people living in smaller spaces and more cars on the streets. In the past few years it has become common to see street trees being cut down because they are considered dangerous;

developers are building ever-smaller homes without gardens or outdoor space; and air-pollution collects on crowded streets.

Most cities, too, are expanding, and their environments are physically degrading. A big survey of European urban areas in 2018 found that the urban surface area of Europe has expanded by a massive 78 per cent since the 1960s, while the population had grown by just one-third. The expansion, which is more than 1,000 square kilometres a year in Europe, has come almost exclusively in the rapidly expanding peri-urban areas – those zones between urban and rural where industry and commerce is now mostly located.

But it is the steady erosion of public, green space that has arguably most affected human health. As if city authorities did not know, the huge health benefits of parks and gardens was seen clearly during the Covid-19 pandemic when public parks offered millions of people their only physical respite from the coronavirus crisis – 'a breathing space amid infection anxieties, crowded flats, home-schooling and job insecurities', as they were described by Rachel Shabi in the *Guardian*. 'With other venues closed, people turned to the nation's 27,000 urban green spaces, from manicured landscapes to patchy neighbourhood parks and playing fields.'[18]

By far the greatest change in the way we live over the past fifty years has been in our reliance on technology and the way people have turned to indoor and virtual recreation and leisure. The 1950s saw the rapid rise of television as the most popular medium of entertainment; video games arrived in the 1970s and the internet has dominated leisure time for the past twenty years. An official UK government study suggests that children in the US, EU, China and most developed countries today spend only half the time their parents did playing outside.[19] Another study, from Seattle, showed that kids aged between ten and sixteen spend fewer than thirteen minutes a day outside, compared to ten waking hours sitting indoors.[20]

Technology, indeed, may be changing the whole human relationship with nature. I spoke to Washington University psychology professor Peter Kahn, who explores how the speed of technological change shapes people and who told me, 'Children come of age watching digital nature programmes on television. They inhabit virtual lands in digital games and they play with robotic animals. They communicate with their friends digitally, they spend seven hours or more a day on screen. They search for knowledge with computers, and they rely on it to see the world.'[21]

> We are a technological species—we've always been one. But for hundreds of thousands of years our technologies were rudimentary. When our minds evolved from palaeolithic to neolithic to now, our technologies did, too. We're drawn to technologies not only because they are foisted on us by corporations, but also because the impetus for them lies within the architecture of our very being. But, even though we are a technological species, we are now out of balance. To thrive, we need more nature and more wild forms of interaction with more wild nature; I doubt we need tons of new technology.[22]

Catharine Ward Thompson, professor of landscape architecture at Edinburgh University and co-author of a World Health Organization report on urban green spaces and health,[23] has brilliantly charted how nature has always been associated with physical and mental health and well-being.[24] In 2011 she reminded us that the old Persian word for enclosed park or orchard, 'pairi-daeza', gave us the word 'paradise', and how cuneiform tablets speak of the gardens of the ancient city of Dilmun, where 'human beings are untouched by illness'.[25]

The restorative health benefits of gardens and the wider landscape have been known and recognised by every culture and age, from the great Greek physicians Galen and Hippocrates through to the Romans and on to Dominicans and medieval monastic orders, she says. *The Epic of Gilgamesh* – often called the first great work of literature – describes how Gilgamesh eventually reaches a healthful, paradise garden of the gods that delights every sense and supports humans in every way. Ward Thompson quotes Pliny the Younger, writing in *c.* AD 100, who had a villa in Laurentum, outside Rome. '"All is calm and composed; which circumstances contribute no less than its clear air and unclouded sky to that health of body and mind I particularly enjoy in this place." '[26]

Her conclusion should be a lesson to any modern authority wanting to nurture a healthy population: 'Loss and degradation of urban green space contributes to the burden of disease, exacerbating the effects of other adverse factors in the urban environment, such as inequalities, air pollution, noise, chronic stress and insufficient physical activity.'[27]

18

HEALING THE LAND

Sabarmatee Apa and her father Radha Mohan knew what they wanted when they tried to buy land in eastern India in 1989. It had to have few trees or vegetation and be without animals or water, and it did not matter if it had been doused in chemicals. It was most important that it was land that no one wanted.

'We wanted land without hope, we wanted the worst possible,' Sabarmatee told me when I first met her.[1] Their idea was to conduct an ecological experiment by taking the most degraded and broken land they could find, regenerating it using no synthetic chemicals and then grow food there for themselves and, if possible, others. They were to start with nothing and to spend nothing. Could it be done? They hoped so, but they knew it might fail or take a lifetime.

It took the duo, who had no great farming background, several years to find the right patch of India, but in 1989 they bought one acre (around 4,000 square metres) of an abandoned former forest in the Nayagarh district of Odisha. It was perfect, a remnant of an ancient, dense forest where tigers once lived, but which had been felled and burned during a famine in the 1940s to provide potassium. The trees had mostly gone, the topsoil had been badly damaged and heavy rains had eroded what was left. It had been heavily farmed for millet with pesticides and herbicides for a few years, but it was as close as it's possible to get to dead land.

Getting to their patch of land from Odisha's capital city, Bhubaneswar, takes all day on crowded roads. Set in hills and forests, it is a centre of stone quarrying and rice farming. Now a middle-aged woman with a wide, ready smile and a calm manner, Sabarmatee has no internet access or telephone, and the duo pick up messages only when they travel to a town. Her father, Radha, was a professor of economics at Odisha University but is now retired and in his seventies. They were both charming and welcoming.

She picks up the story. 'It was hard at first. We had no running water, we slept in the open. We started by rebuilding the soil and collecting the water. We stacked up leaves and waste and allowed them to decay. After three years, the results slowly became visible. To start with, the land was covered in lush green grass which encouraged insects. Gradually, it became topsoil that was cultivable with heavy mulching. 'We wanted to prove a point how ecology can be restored in a totally degraded land without the use of external inputs including fertilisers and pesticides. We have followed ecological principles only,' said Radha.

They brought in grasses and planted mangoes and bamboo, and other trees to stop the soil erosion. Healing the soil was the greatest challenge, Sabarmatee says. 'We protected the plants that came up on their own and we mulched and mulched. Eventually the worms came, the ants, the millipedes, the spiders, butterflies, bees, and other pollinators. Then the bigger life started to come back. The wild boar, birds, snakes and insects. We learned that life supports life. The trees brought the birds, the dragonflies and butterflies. The most important work was done by the birds. Thousands of birds came,' said Sabarmatee.

Bit by bit they added more land and kept planting, mulching and collecting seeds, constructing an elaborate system of ponds and water collecting. 'Everyone was very discouraging at first. They made fun of us and said we were crazy. First they said we could not grow trees on it, then they said we could not grow crops there, then that we could not grow rice. Eventually they came and together we have shown what can be done.'

Today the father-daughter duo call their thirty years on this once blasted land 'a journey from the impossible ("asambhav" in Hindi) to the possible ("sambhav")'. What started as a small patch of wasteland is now a lush 40-hectare 'food forest' with almost a hectare of nearly 500 varieties of rice, a wealth of mango, lychees and coconut trees, an elaborate system of rainwater harvesting ponds, and more than a thousand species of plants. At the heart of it all is a sanctuary where indigenous varieties of rice and other plants are grown for their seeds, which are then exchanged. Their edible forest is now worked and used by the local community. Farmers come to help and be trained. 'Human health and the health of the land? It is the same thing for us,' says Sabarmatee.

'We journeyed from the impossible to the possible. My father and I never believed this to be a wasteland. But, it was being wasted. We planted where there was nothing. Yes, we had doubts sometimes. Now I believe there is no such thing as waste land, only wasted land. It doesn't need science to give life to land. Give me one grain and I can give you ten kilograms in a few years. There's magic in a handful of seeds. Unless we take care of nature we will have no hope. If we look after it, the land will heal and we will be healthy too.'

She laughed out loud. 'But we don't want the tiger back. Everyone will flee.'

* * *

Restoring degraded land is not difficult. It can be as simple as changing farming methods or leaving land to lie fallow, saving water, planting different crops or regrowing trees to stop soils blowing away. Sabarmatee and her father's initiative in Odisha is just one of many thousands of inspirational efforts to heal damaged land, now taking place at different scales in nearly every country. They show that it is nearly always possible to restore human, animal and plant health. They are beacons for the future. By taking land that seems beyond hope and making it healthy again, they suggest that a revolution in human, animal and plant health is both possible and underway.

But the task is enormous. Quite how much land has been severely damaged in the past centuries is startling. In its 2018 report on climate change and land, the UN estimates it could be as much as 60 million square kilometres – an area about twice the size of China. Another study suggests that one-third of the Earth's land surface is degraded, affecting more than 2.6 billion people.[2] Restoring it is essential to feed people and improve human and animal health, as well as counter climate change and lower temperatures.

Brazilian economist and social scientist Bernardo Strassburg links the large-scale restoration of degraded land to planetary health. With colleagues from Brazil, Australia and Europe, he led a major study in 2018 to identify how much land could be restored and where in the world it would be best to concentrate efforts. He was astonished. 'If a third of the planet's most degraded areas were planted with trees and restored to ecological health, and protection was thrown around those areas still in good condition, half of all human caused greenhouse gas emissions emitted since the industrial revolution would be captured,' Strassburg told me.[3]

Land restoration takes many forms, from small-scale 'rewilding' projects with the emphasis on humans stepping back and leaving areas to recover on their own, to more active management where ecosystems are upgraded with new species of plants and animals and trees are planted on a large scale. Some projects are conservation-led and intended to return cultivated land to a more natural state for the sake of biodiversity, often reintroducing lost species, and removing alien species and damaging infrastructure such as dams. Others, like Sabarmatee and her father's project in India, involve human intervention and are intended to both grow food and heal the environment.

Rewilding projects that allow nature to run wild are now springing up everywhere, led in the UK and other parts of Europe by large estate owners. Some, like that at Knepp Castle in southern England, where 800 hectares of low-grade farmland have been allowed to grow unhindered by humans since 2001, appear passive but aim to make considerable profits through tourism. In the Netherlands an area of reclaimed polder land called the Oostvaardersplassen has for forty years been restoring the Dutch landscape to much as it was before humans began intensively cultivating it. This pioneering project became controversial when hundreds of animals died in a bitter winter when humans did not intervene.

At the other end of the spectrum are megaprojects intended by governments and international bodies to restore entire damaged and degraded landscapes, mostly with massive tree-planting schemes. As of 2022, there are national campaigns to plant many billions of trees. Saudi Arabia has pledged to plant 10 billion, Africa 100 million. Pakistan hit its target of planting 1 billion trees and has set a new target of 10 billion by 2025. China plans to green the Gobi Desert and extend and conserve its forests. In 2017, 1.5 million Indian volunteers planted 66 million trees in twelve hours in Madhya Pradesh. India says it will increase its forests by 95 million hectares by 2030. Africa plans to bring 100 million hectares of land into restoration by 2030.

Tim Christopherson, the UN's environment, climate and nature head, says an area the size of China needs to recover. For that to happen, restoration needs to be seen as a global infrastructure priority, on the level of space exploration, or as important as roads and ports. 'For many people, I think restoring a billion hectares is abstract. [But] we have decades of experience of how this could work but never on the scale we're talking about. We have space programmes and nuclear weapons – it is possible.'[4]

Planting trees makes instinctive sense. It appears cheap, easy to understand and is mostly popular. Trees, after all, diminish flood risk, improve air quality by absorbing pollution and yield a renewable resource. They can reduce soil degradation on farms and provide vital habitat for wildlife, as well as food, fuel and medicine. Most importantly, in the climate emergency, trees sequester carbon. Trees mitigate climate change and tree planting is now recognised as one of the best ways to tackle this global crisis.

Dozens of national and international targets, initiatives and challenges have been set. The UN Environment programme wants governments to commit to restore 3.5 million square kilometres of land over the coming decade – slightly more than the size of India, or just over 2 per cent of the world's land surface. The Bonn

Challenge, set up by Germany and the UN, calls for the restoration of 350 million hectares by 2030, while the Sustainable Development Goals go further still, aiming for land degradation neutrality by 2030. The combined ambition is staggering. According to the UN, it might cost $1 trillion but the health and economic benefits of what would be the fastest reshaping of earth's surface by any species are incalculable.

A grand start has been made. When in 2019 Annelies Sewell at the Dutch government's Environmental Assessment Agency totted up the existing commitments to land restoration projects she found they added up to more than 10 million square kilometres in 115 countries, with countries pledging to increase protected areas, restore and improve forests, croplands and grasslands, and more. 'There's more than we expected,' says Sewell.[5]

Africa, so often cast as the laggard in environmental affairs, has led the way. An old Africa Union vision has been revived of an 8,000-kilometre-long, fifteen-kilometre-wide belt of trees and farmland covering 100 million hectares. It would snake through eleven countries bordering the southern Sahara Desert from Senegal in the west of the continent to Djibouti in the east.

'The Great Green Wall', as it is dubbed, would not be a solid wall of trees so much as a necklace of farmland and forestry with croplands and pastures set in and among tree plantations, nurseries, grasslands, fruit orchards and villages. Yes, it would conserve biodiversity, but its strength is in the recognition that human health and well-being is directly linked to, and dependent on, the state of health of the ecosystems that support them.

Inspired partly by colonial ecologist and forester Richard St Barbe Baker, who spent the 1920s in Africa as a conservator of forests, the Green Wall plan is intended not just to hold back the desert, but to improve nutrition and health for millions of people living in some of the world's fastest-growing and hungriest countries.

Barker was a pioneer conservationist, an eccentric who worked tirelessly to protect forests and, through observation, proved that the Sahara Desert was once wooded. From 1945 onwards he pestered governments and lobbied relentlessly for the world's armies to plant 'a green wall' to avoid an ecological collapse engulfing much of Africa. Way ahead of his time, he recommended in the 1960s that China send troops into the Gobi to plant trees to hold back the desert. Work began in 1978 with farmers and in 2017 the Chinese government reportedly sent a regiment of the People's Liberation Army to complete the planting of 6.6 million hectares – an area nearly the size of Ireland.[6]

Now backed by the Africa Union, the UN and the World Bank, the Great Green Wall is one of the world's most inspirational projects,[7] harnessing money and enthusiasm across Africa. The dryland borders of the Sahel are the frontline of climate change, close to being too hot and degraded for people or animals to live there but still possible to restore. Not only is the 'wall' expected to provide jobs and improve health in one of the poorest regions of the world, but it could sequester 250 million tonnes of carbon in a volatile, vulnerable environment.

Already quiet revolutions, barely registering in the West, are taking place along its route. Since the middle of the 1980s, smallholder farmers in densely populated parts of Niger, the fastest-growing country in the world, have begun to protect and manage woody species which regenerated spontaneously on their farmland. Over 200 million trees have been planted and 5 million hectares of degraded land 're-greened' in Niger.

The result, says a report by global agricultural research centre IFPRI (the International Food Policy Research Institute), has been an extra 500,000 tonnes of food grown in the country, as well as an increase in biodiversity and incomes. In Burkina Faso, where 200,000–300,000 hectares of land has been regenerated, food production has grown about 80,000 tonnes a year – enough to feed an extra 500,000 people.[8]

* * *

One woman may be said to have kickstarted the modern land restoration revolution. Wangari Maathai, who grew up in a modest family home in a village in the foothills of the Aberdare mountains in central Kenya, had excelled at school, won a scholarship to study in the US and was working as a biologist and a vet at the University of Kenya. But it was when researching ticks in cattle that she saw that the rivers she had known as a child, which had then been clear, were now filled with silt. The cattle were skinny and people were emaciated.

It was so different from her childhood. When growing up in the 1940s, hunger and disease were rare in the Central Highlands of Kenya. In those days the community grew cassava, sweet potatoes, arrowroots and perennial food crops like bananas and sugar cane, an enormous diversity of foods to cushion people during droughts and crop failures.

But in the intervening years, people had been persuaded by successive governments and colonial authorities to cut down the trees to grow cash crops like tea and coffee for export. The trees, along with the wild fruit and vegetables which they had enjoyed, were gone and so was fresh water. The land looked lush with tea, but it was depleted and the people were malnourished.

I met Wangari first in London in 1989, and then several times in Nairobi. She recalled how it shocked her deeply to see unhealthy people living in such a fertile land and led her to give up university and start the Green Belt movement of women to fight for restoration of the land.

> I talked with my colleagues. We could either sit in an ivory tower wondering why so many people could be so poor and ill or we could try to help them escape the vicious cycle they found themselves in. These were not remote places. This is where our mothers and sisters lived. We owed it to them; the connection between the symptoms of degradation, its deforestation and soil loss were self-evident. We had to get to the cause of the problems. It just came to me. Why not plant trees?[9]

Women, especially, responded to Wangari's suggestion, and in the following decades she mobilised hundreds of communities to plant around 47 million trees. But tree planting and the protection of nature was political. 'The simple act of planting trees challenged the authorities, delivered a rebuke to corrupt and oppressive leaders whose pursuit of power and riches made them indifferent to the starvation and ill-health of their own people,' she said.[10]

Soon after she won the Nobel Peace Prize in 2004, we travelled together from Nairobi to her village of Ihithe, near Nyeri in the foothills of the Aberdare mountains. The family home, where her sister lived, nestled in a deep valley. 'Mother lies there,' she said, quietly. 'My relatives live there. It's heaven. But people there do not appreciate it because we have a political and economic system that does not allow people to appreciate the beauty of where they live. That's the tragedy of poverty.'[11]

The changes that have taken place in Ihithe since the 1950s reflect the linked environmental and health crises which she said were burdening so much of Kenya and the rest of Africa. 'I have seen huge changes. The population has grown enormously. All this area [around Ihithe] was wooded. There were small farms, full of maize, millet and sorghum. The rivers were huge and clean. There was no tea. Today we see tea, tea, tea. Mother never planted tea. Tea has become slave labour. Farming has become the production of a commodity which people cannot process or eat. You cannot process your own tea. Tea without good governance is serfdom and only leads to environmental and health problems.'[12]

Trees, she said, bring health to communities. 'They not only bind the soil, halt erosion and retain groundwater following rains, which in turn replenishes streams, but provide food, fodder, and fuel. They bind the soil together but also communities and give them health. They maintain livelihoods, which ensures health. A degraded environment leads to a scramble for scarce resources which often culminate in poverty and ill-health.'[13]

The tree is just a symbol for what happens to the environment, said Wangari, adding: 'The act of planting one is a symbol of revitalising the community. Tree planting is only the entry point into the wider debate about the environment and health. Everyone should plant a tree.'[14]

* * *

So what can go wrong with tree planting? Plenty. In the rush to plant large areas, serious mistakes are being made. Far from being 'forests for people' or 'climate', as many projects are billed, large-scale tree-planting schemes are often no more than palm oil plantations or eucalyptus forests planted on former tropical forest lands to supply the voracious global pulp paper and palm oil industries and enable countries to meet their carbon targets. Moreover, most will be felled in a few years before they can have any climate or ecological benefit. As is common with so many large projects, large-scale tree planting goes hand in hand with corruption and bad management and often has a very low success rate.

British environmentalist Chris Lang is an assiduous watchdog of the global forestry industry and large-scale tree planting. Too often, he says, the most grandiose-sounding schemes are little more than 'tree-washing'. 'There is a tendency to assume that green is good, and that green is fair. Many projects involve get-rich-quick scams for carbon capture, corruption and land-grabs,' says Lang.[15]

Some forests are planted in the wrong place and die within months; others are prone to disease or are unsuitable for the climate. 'Active restoration brings risks if done badly,' adds Bernardo Strassburg. 'Any scaled-up restoration needs to be ecologically sound. It is not just planting trees everywhere, particularly in places where trees didn't belong in the first place.'[16]

Grassland experts are appalled. From a climate perspective, planting mega forests across swathes of grass makes little sense. Not only has grassland, which covers most of the land not covered by trees, been found to fix carbon and be more reliable than trees, but it can reflect solar radiation better than dark forests, even cooling the earth.[17]

Just as worryingly, the scale of planting envisaged almost certainly means that hundreds of thousands of people in relatively poor countries will be evicted from their farmland to make way for trees. Industrial tree plantations almost always involve human rights abuses, exclude people, livestock and wildlife, and result in less biodiversity.[18]

* * *

Even as Sabarmatee and her father started to mulch the land in India in 1989, far-seeing but anonymous civil servants were putting forward to the British government the idea of planting what they called 'a new national forest'. Britain, they reasoned, had 1,000 years ago been densely forested but generations of urbanisation, population growth, quarrying, shipbuilding and, especially, coal mining had devastated landscapes and tree cover had reduced to less than 13 per cent of the land – by some way the lowest of any G7 country.[19] Now, with heavy industry almost gone, they said, it was the time to plant.

It took years for the penny-pinching, ecologically illiterate central government to do anything, but, stung by accusations that it was telling developing countries like Brazil not to cut down their trees while having cut down nearly all of theirs, they agreed. The old South Derbyshire coalfield in the English Midlands was chosen as an experiment.

When I first visited the area in 1993 just before work on the forest was to start, I was shocked. It was a miserable, cold March morning and I had seldom seen such a grim landscape. The villages of Moira, Donisthorpe and Overseal were surrounded by open-cast mines, old clay quarries, spoil heaps, derelict coal workings, polluted waterways and all the other ecological wreckage of redundant heavy industry. The air smelled stale and tasted sulphurous, and the soils were coal-black and poisoned. There were next to no trees, few jobs and very little wildlife. Following the closure of the coal pits, I was told, people were deserting the area for cities such as Birmingham, Derby and Leicester.

I returned twenty-five years later and recognised nothing. A genuine social and ecological renaissance had taken place in what was the broken heart of the coalfield. In place of the slag, or spoil, tips and the degraded land, a vast young oak, ash and birch forest was emerging, attracting cyclists, walkers, birdwatchers, canoeists, campers and horse-riders. A charity had taken over many of the area's old industrial workings and was advising landowners and farmers about switching from low-grade farmland to forest and woodland.

With little fuss, more than 9 million trees had been planted, hundreds of kilometres of footpath created and nearly 500 abandoned industrial sites had been made safe and transformed, all for under £5 million of government money – a pittance which might build a few hundred metres of new motorway. The landscape and ecology of a significant part of semi-derelict Britain has been revived and rewilded with trees in a single generation. It was not a dense, closed canopy forest but a mosaic of farmland, woods and lakes. Today, property there is sought after, and more than 4 million visitors a year from surrounding towns visit the forest to picnic, walk, play sports and appreciate the new landscape.

The health benefits of the ecological transformation that has taken place have not been rigorously quantified, but everyone I spoke to was adamant that their lives were healthier. Graham Knight, a former coalface engineer who now worked for a charity which was retraining people to work again, put it well: 'This was clay pits, quarries, coal mines, chimneys, sewer pipes and kilns. It was very unhealthy, pretty grim. It was a hard life and it toughened people up. The area went into steep decline when the industry closed and almost everything disappeared. It has changed from a wasteland to an environment that we envied. People love trees, don't they? They like to see forests and woods. In those days you would not go to a place like this for holidays. People are moving in and communities are now growing.'[20]

It was not only human health that had improved, he said. Along with the maturing trees had come buzzards and red kites, skylarks, butterflies, otters, bats and owls. As the trees grew, insects and small mammals came too. John Everitt, director of the National Forest Company, which ran the forest, was proud of the changes. 'This is one of the largest landscape transformations in the United Kingdom, the first major forest to have been planted in England for a thousand years. We have taken a black hole and given it a new lease of life; given people a new landscape. We can say that air pollution is better, people are healthier, the rivers are cleaner, the water is being retained better and soil is being better conserved.'[21]

I called at random two medical surgeries in the district and asked to speak to the doctor or health worker who had practised there the longest. I had just one question: had health improved since coal mining had ended and the land had been restored? I got one quick answer from everyone: 'Yes.'

* * *

But even the most ambitious schemes can be knocked off course. I saw this in Tigray, in northern Ethiopia, where sparse, steep and rocky soils have always made farming precarious. Here the rains may last a month or two at best and temperatures can climb to well over 40°C. In the 1980s the province was at the epicentre of one of the worst famines of the past hundred years, when successive droughts crippled farming, tens of thousands of people died and millions more fled or were left dependent on foreign aid. Plagues of locusts destroyed crops in 2020 and in November 2020 the Eritrean and the Ethiopian government armies invaded.

Tigray faces all the world's great ecological problems – climate change, rising temperatures, degraded lands, water shortages, conflict, hunger, insecurity and deep poverty. But until war with the central government broke out in November 2020, it was gaining the reputation of being a place where people were overcoming environmental disaster.

Forty years ago villages around Abrha Weatsbha were close to being abandoned. The hillsides were barren, the land was blighted and communities were plagued by floods and deep droughts. Constant food aid was needed, ill health was rife and the soil was being washed away, and people were leaving to live in poverty in cities. It was a catastrophic failure of the environment.

What happened in the intervening years was little short of miraculous. Rather than just plant trees, which is notoriously unreliable and expensive in dryland areas, villagers in the early 1990s were encouraged to turn to 'agro-ecology', a way to combine crops and trees on the same pieces of land.

It was a regeneration project on a grand scale. Terraces were constructed, percolation trenches dug to replenish the groundwater and mini dams built to hold back every drop of water. Large areas of land were closed off to animals to allow the natural regeneration of trees and vegetation and the widespread planting of seedlings. Within ten years the results could be seen. According to researchers, hillsides were green again, and natural springs that had dried up started to flow. Whole mountainsides had been terraced, and on the lower slopes irrigated fields. Numerous individual wells and ponds were full of water. The saving of water allowed hundreds of shallow wells to be dug and high-value vegetable crops to be grown. Villagers were in better health, able to harvest vegetables, fruit and maize even in the dry season.

By 2019 significant parts of Tigray were greener than they had been in almost 150 years, not because rainfall had increased, but because land restoration was working. 'The people ... may have moved more earth and stone [in recent years] to reshape the surface of their land than the Egyptians during thousands of years to build the pyramids,' said Chris Reij, a land specialist and a researcher with the World Resources Institute in Washington. For a while, the social and health benefits of this agro-ecological approach cascaded down. 'People eat better, drink better, are happier, wealthier and healthier. It's win-win-win, one of the biggest and best news stories of the decade,' he told me enthusiastically.[22]

But war trumps everything. By the summer of 2021, reports confirmed that the many ecological gains made were being lost as young men left to become fighters. Oxen, used to plough farmlands, had been deliberately killed by invading Ethiopian and Eritrean soldiers. There was hardly any access to seed.

I spoke again with Reij in 2021. He was distraught. All the restoration and re-greening work was likely to be reversed and another famine was likely. It was a disaster that would take another generation to recover from, he said.[23]

* * *

I could see how human and animal health could be improved by restoration and tree planting, but I wanted to see if land that had been used for large-scale cereal farming could also be transformed to both improve social conditions and increase food production. This time I travelled to the village of Foros de Vale de Figueira in southern Portugal, where I had been told of an agroforestry experiment – farming with trees.

Thousands of hectares around the village had been farmed over centuries by Romans, Moors, Christians, capitalists, far rightists, even the military. It had been part of a private fiefdom and worked by slaves as well as communists. Some of the great old Portuguese cork oak forest remained but much of the land was now an empty grassland without people or animals, wilting under a baking Iberian sun. Droughts and higher temperatures had made the soil prone to erosion and the terrain to forest fires.

The estate was being farmed by Alfredo Cunhal Sendim, who had trained as an agricultural scientist. His great-grandfather had cleared many of the ancient cork and olive trees and generations of relatives had then overworked the land by dosing it with chemicals and growing vast hectares of cereals. Cunhal had been expected to carry on, reaping large but short-term profits.

> I had to reject much of what I was taught about farming at college. I spent five years studying agriculture and I never heard the word ecology. We were taking more and more from the land but we were farming monocultures. We were eating the system. I was managing 7,000 hectares for my family but I never noticed the trees. I really didn't know anything. I produced a lot but I needed so many inputs. I needed carbon, energy, and chemicals. I could do nothing efficiently. The land was eroded, the soil damaged.[24]

Demoralised, unwell and depressed, he gave up managing the family estate in 1990, took a share of his family's land, and started to run 600 hectares on organic, cooperative lines with a collective of thirty-five people, many of whom had worked on the estate for years. Together, he and his 'partners' were now converting the whole farm into a full *montado* system – a pre-medieval Portuguese way of farming which combined herds of animals with productive trees and shrubs. Their vision was to create an oasis-style abundance on land where there is often no rain for nine months of the year and where temperatures can reach 49°C.

His vision is utterly different from his family's. We sat under a 2,000-year-old olive tree as he outlined the ecological transformation of the land to provide food and good human and animal health. 'Monocultures and specialisation are the end of life. Resilience and safety comes in diversity. This is real human health.'

> Imagine tall trees, like forty-metre-tall walnuts, letting light through, drawing up water. Below them, cork oaks giving shade, and a line of citrus and olive trees; and then imagine vines climbing the trees. The fruit and nuts will provide the food for the pigs, chickens, cows and other animals who graze there.

Cunhal said he had always instinctively understood that human, animal and plant health were interlinked but had not made the practical connections. Now he was certain.

> Animals are the key. They are important for the whole ecosystem, as well as part of the food chain. They must be balanced with the tree system. Pigs provide digestion, and are good for the soil, they disturb the ground and fertilise the land. The natural fertility cycles work better with them. The pig is not a meat machine but a friend of nature and humans. We are aiming to go from zero to abundance in a few years. We can put chickens on the land soon, pigs and sheep will follow, cows come later. We invest now, and the next generation sees the real benefits of health.[25]

The results were beginning to show. They had so far planted nearly 40,000 oaks and other trees, and wild boar, lynx and deer had returned. Old varieties of pig, cattle, chickens and turkeys were being rotated among the established oak and olive trees and in newly planted orchards. The farm was growing almost every type of Mediterranean food among the trees, as well as forty varieties of fruit and nuts, and selling 600 different products ranging from eight kinds of oak flour and breads to meat, wine and olive oil. Now it was also a living laboratory where more than a thousand different species of animal and plant had been recorded.

There was nothing that could not grow, even in such a hot climate, said Cunhal. 'We can even grow water. By planting trees whose roots go deep we are drawing moisture up and building soils; we create the possibility to grow even more.'

* * *

I found Luwayo Biswick's five-acre permaculture farm in central Malawi thanks to two young Americans who had gone to Malawi nearly twenty years before to help with the HIV crisis. Stacia Nordin, a registered dietician, and Kristof, a social worker, had been US Peace Corps volunteers and had quickly learned that the Southern African country had some of the highest malnutrition[26] and HIV/Aids levels[27] in the world, and that modern drugs alone were not the answer.

Poverty, poor health and limited diets go together in Malawi, where, thanks to British colonial advice, farming is overwhelmingly focused on growing maize, a staple crop which is easy enough to grow in good times, but is vulnerable to droughts, heatwaves, floods and insect infestations.[28] The result is that malnutrition is rife and most people remain desperately poor. With climate change, malaria, dengue and other zoonotic diseases are common.

'Poor nutrition contributes to the progression of HIV,' Stacia told me. 'We couldn't address a disease that attacks the immune system without addressing the fact that immune systems are compromised by malnutrition. We couldn't work on improving nutrition without working to improve the diversity of what was being grown. And we couldn't improve the diversity of agricultural crops without working to improve soil fertility.'[29]

Together the couple learned to farm by observing how nature works, meeting people and experimenting. Within fifteen years of buying a one-hectare, average-size Malawian peasant smallholding, they had transformed it into a Garden of Eden by mimicking the many levels of a forest, mulching, composting, collecting rainwater and planting crops close together.

When I met them in 2015, the Nordins were growing more than fifty local foods, collecting their own seeds, and teaching nutrition and permaculture to government officials, church leaders, schools and other farmers. Mango trees grew beside tall tamarinds, acacia, guavas, passion fruit and coconut palms. Below them were lemon and orange trees, tomatoes, blackjack, maize and cassava. The ground was thick with pineapples and watermelon, and decomposing leaves and other plants covered a rich soil growing yams and sweet potatoes.

But they had also trained Luwayo Biswick, a young Malawian. After five years he had left to set up his own farm sixty kilometres away. It, too, was a food forest and the contrast between it and the lands beyond his property was stark. Where he was growing fifty crops and had a ten-month growing season, picking fresh fruit and vegetables throughout the year, most farmers were growing only maize. He now teaches people from all over Africa how to achieve extraordinary yields by planting a huge diversity of foods in very small areas, without using chemical fertilisers, pesticides or mechanisation.

Biswick calls his project 'Paradise Permaculture' for good reason.

In just three years we managed to transform a dead land; the soil was sandy and depleted. The previous owner used to monocrop the land so there was very little life in it and very little diversity. Feeding and improving the soil definitely has helped improve human and plant health. Most land in Malawi is dry and dusty, which leads to bronchial problems and human diseases and infections. During the Covid-19 pandemic we had no problems with flu and coughs, as compared to others who had a lot of problems. We also noted that our soils absorb water quickly; there is no standing water, hence no mosquito breeding areas and no malaria. In short, I would say there is a very strong connection between soil and human health.[30]

The abiding narrative of many Western conservationists these last twenty years has been that nature is fragile, diseased and on the brink of collapse. But the reality, seen now in thousands of places and projects, is that when given a chance, it is infinitely resilient and well able to recover quickly from almost any human abuse. Far from being interlopers in the natural world, humans are amazingly powerful ecosystem engineers, and potential forces of good health for all life.

CONCLUSION: NATURE FIRST AND LAST

Ye can call it influenza if you like. There was no influenza in
my day. We called a cold a cold.

Arnold Bennett, *The Card*, 1911

The small Canadian city of Merritt in British Columbia looked
like a bomb had hit it after nearly thirty centimetres of rain fell
in a few hours and the Coldwater river broke its banks and raged
through its streets on the weekend of 13 November 2021. Bridges
were submerged, buildings were ripped from their foundations,
cars lay crumpled, trees were uprooted and 5,000 people had to be
hurriedly evacuated.

But it was when the flood had subsided and people started
to return to what was left of their city that the connection was
made between this 'natural' disaster and a series of other seemingly
random events that had affected the wider region months before.
Back in July and August 2021, British Columbia had experienced
an unprecedented, blistering heatwave which had left the state's
great forests tinder-dry. Uncontrolled wildfires followed and nearly
8,700 square kilometres of forest, as well as the whole town of
Lytton, just a one hour's drive from Merritt, burned to the ground.

Climatologists quickly attributed the heatwave and fires to
climate change but, unnoticed at the time, the forest soils had

baked hard in the heat, making them water-repellent. So when the torrential rains came in November, the water rushed off the steep slopes faster than usual and caused land- and mudslides. Sediment diverted rivers, causing floods often hundreds of kilometres away in places like Merritt that had never known them before. It was a compound climate disaster.

What happened at Merritt was more than a reminder of the perils of climate change. The floods also overwhelmed the city's sewage plant as well as many residents' septic tanks. Cellars and living rooms were filled with contaminated water sometimes containing the decomposing bodies of animals and the pathogens which cause diarrhoeal diseases, vomiting and fevers.

In short, planetary change led to local change (fire) which led to a third change (flood) which created the conditions for a fourth change (disease). Learning how ecological disruption works on many scales and cascades down must now be a priority of the age.

* * *

When I first went to Gabon in 2004 to investigate a small Ebola outbreak on the edge of the great Minkebe forest, governments, physicians, journalists and researchers barely guessed that deforestation or gold mining, factory farming or indeed climate change might give rise to new human diseases. That has changed thanks to the detective work done by virologists and epidemiologists and to far greater knowledge about the forces that change the global environment.

But what have we really learned since 2004? We know from bitter experience that infectious diseases can now spread everywhere, bringing death and misery to hundreds of millions of people in a very short time. We know, too, that they are becoming more common. Covid-19 has taught us that the emergence of disease is mostly driven by environmental change. Unless there is a fundamental rethink about how we coexist with nature, then pandemics will recur more frequently.

Covid-19 has mostly shocked those wealthy countries that imagined they were immune to the pandemics and disease outbreaks that less developed ones must endure regularly. As well as the continuing pandemic of HIV/Aids, in twenty years there have been many other, less serious human and animal ones that have gone largely unnoticed by the international media either because they have not impacted much in the West, or because they have been more or less constrained and therefore less newsworthy.

But we now see that rich countries in temperate regions like the EU and North America had dodged many bullets until Covid-19 arrived. Nipah was mostly confined to Thailand, SARS to South Asia, MERS to Saudi Arabia and Zika to Latin America. Equally, H1N1 swine flu was mostly mild, H5N1 was largely confined to poultry and Hendra burned out in Australia. Meanwhile, diseases like Mpox, CJD, BSE, West Nile virus and Bolivian hemorrhagic fever – any of which in the right circumstances could have spread around the world – have mercifully not spread far. In retrospect, only extraordinary work by vets, physicians, ecologists and others has prevented more catastrophic diseases from emerging and spreading in the last twenty years.

Looking back, we can also see that most of these diseases did not just happen because of weak health systems, globalisation and inequality, but were ecologically driven and human-made in the sense that our lifestyles and consumption patterns have created the ideal physical conditions for them to thrive. By altering the planetary environment and changing the local ecological conditions in which we and other species live, by coming closer to animals and living closer together in cities, we have been providing microbes perfect conditions in which to evolve and mutate faster, and in which they are more likely to jump species.[1]

Nor were these many diseases unexpected. Animals, especially, have played a major part in nearly every major disease outbreak since 2004, via markets, the wildlife trade, deforestation, laboratory experiments, the vast global poultry, pig and pet industries and the unsanitary conditions that people must endure in some urban areas. It is more than likely that the next great pandemic, just like Covid-19, will be a novel virus that crosses to humans from an animal.

But we should not despair. There have been astonishing discoveries and developments. In under twenty years we have learned far more about how microorganisms work; how ecosystems respond to global environmental changes; how climate change is altering geographic boundaries and affecting human, animal and plant health, and will do so far more in future. We know how to make better vaccines faster, and we can tell now when an ecosystem is near a tipping point. We know how to treat disease better and how to monitor and analyse virus variants faster.

We have come a long way in just twenty years but the uncertainties have only mounted. We do not know exactly how – or even when or where – any of these twenty-first-century pandemics and outbreaks started, except that each one has been connected to the way humans have changed physical environments, be it by fire, flood, animal farming, logging, or, increasingly, by degrading land, deforestation and climate change. There is no general mechanistic theory of global environmental change and emerging disease. But twenty years of investigation and mounting empirical evidence shows that human, plant and animal illnesses are inextricably linked to the health of the environment and how humans shape it. We may have no idea how dangerous any new virus or mutation of an existing one may be; nor do we know whether it will attack the very young, the old or everyone, how severe or transmissible it may be, which group of animals it will come from, how long it will last, how it may switch to humans, or what will make it mutate. We can be pretty sure, however, that it will impact the poorest hardest, and that it is just as likely to come from North America or Europe as Africa or Asia.

The sobering truth is that we are only inching towards understanding the web of life that binds people, animals, plants and other living organisms to each other and to greater planetary systems like climate, atmosphere and ocean currents. We suspect that there may be 10,000 unidentified species of virus in animals with the potential to spread in human populations, yet only a few hundred zoonotic viruses are known and many groups of them are woefully understudied.[2]

But we do know that the very short period between 2004 and 2022 has seen some of the fastest-ever transformations of the world's forests, wetlands and soils to provide food, as well as the greatest mining and extraction of fossil fuels for energy, power and minerals, and the biggest increase ever known in trade and human travel.[3] We have never farmed so many animals so intensively, fragmented so many ecosystems, experimented with so many genes or pathogens, or polluted soils, water and the atmosphere so much. Changing climate and land use are already driving geographic range shifts in wildlife, producing novel species assemblages and opportunities for viral sharing between previously isolated species. The connection between our actions and the diseases that humans, animals and plants have suffered have followed as night follows day.

We should have learned that infectious diseases now bring as much misery as war. Since 2004, around 1 million people have died in battle, but at least 50 million have died from infectious diseases.[4] We should also have learned that diseases of the environment are mostly those of the poor. From air pollution, which affects hundreds of millions of people everywhere on earth, to TB, Zika, Covid-19, HIV/Aids and malaria, infectious diseases are more likely to be found in poor cities and areas of major environmental change.

Since 2004, too, we have learned that there is no escape from infectious disease. Borders can be closed for a while, travel restricted and tests demanded of travellers, but viruses and their variants are unstoppable if they have enough hosts. Since 2004, the global supply chains have become even more integrated, and travel is faster, making it even easier for microbes to hitch a ride around the world. Today we share the same diseases. A virus in one country is now more likely than even twenty years ago to reach another and infect everyone.

Outbreaks, epidemics and pandemics are a fact of nature. But that does not mean that we are helpless in their face. We have learned that avoiding infectious disease is far more efficient than scrambling to come up with plans and vaccines after one arrives. Covid-19 is thought to have already cost $11 trillion,[5] SARS cost Southeast Asia at least $50 billion, MERS cost South Korea around

$10 billion,[6] Zika nearly killed the Caribbean tourist industry and Ebola reduced the Sierra Leone and Liberian economies by 10 per cent. A single year of a major bird flu pandemic is forecast to cost $800 billion[7] and even without Covid, infectious diseases may already be costing governments $500 billion a year – one-third of the $1.5 trillion spent a year on defence by the world's rich countries and far more than the world spends on education or poverty alleviation.[8] Future historians may justifiably conclude that humanity's real adversary in the twenty-first century was the microbe. Governments are spending trillions of dollars annually on military defence, but a fraction of that on avoiding, preparing, controlling or treating infectious diseases, even though they inflict far more deaths and much greater economic damage on societies than modern warfare.

One major 2018 study calculates that it would cost in the region of only $3 billion to develop new vaccines for eleven of the world's most infectious diseases, including chikungunya, Zika, Rift Valley fever, MRS and Marburg.[9] The fault lies as much with governments' reluctance to invest as it does in the major vaccine companies, who balk at investing up to $500 million in developing a vaccine for a disease that may not strike rich people or derive them profit.

Reassuringly, we do know that vaccines have improved. Fast-developing mRNA technology may lead to better flu vaccines that could be updated quickly, even the development of a 'universal' flu shot that might be effective for several years. One of the biggest lessons we've learned is that the scientific community working together can do some pretty amazing things. In the past it's taken between four and twenty years to create conventional vaccines. The new messenger RNA (mRNA) vaccines take just eleven months.

But Covid-19 has also taught the world that lasting good health depends on a good relationship with nature, and that medical inventiveness, while brilliant, is not a cure. A global pandemic requires everyone to be immunised, because the longer a virus continues to spread unchecked anywhere in the world in an unvaccinated population, the more likely it is that a variant that can overcome a vaccine will emerge and mutate, putting everyone back to square one. When only people in rich countries are immunised, the number of cases in the world will increase and a novel virus will have more opportunities to mutate and will inevitably find a way through the best defence. Equally, the more we use antibiotics, the more microorganisms will learn to adapt to them and we will need new ones.

In short, if we do not address the cause of disease, rather than try to treat it with vaccines, we are in danger of making infectious diseases stronger at the same time as making ourselves weaker. The only way to ensure good long-term planetary or human health is to bear down on viruses hard and fast, but better by far is to prevent diseases occurring by minimising the disturbance of nature and the interactions between ourselves and the pathogens of other species. The health and environment crises are twins.

* * *

Back in 2004, when I was in the Gabon forests, there was a lingering belief that infectious disease could be controlled by treating the sick and vaccinating people or animals who are at risk. We still hope that fast-developing technologies will lead to better vaccines and that improved drugs will help us avoid the worst illnesses, but we have more or less ignored the causes of disease. There was little incentive to address nature because we could barely understand how it affected human health or wealth and little research was being done to show how our treatment of the planet and disease were linked. No one anticipated the onslaught of emerging infectious diseases that are confronting humans today.[10]

Infectious diseases are part of our evolutionary story and will continue to break out, mutate and haunt us. But whom they affect and where they strike depends entirely on us and is increasingly predictable. Human health today is linked, as ever, to wealth, geography and people's living conditions, but the well-being of humanity now depends on how we choose to live with other species. Knowing that we are at extreme risk warns us of what will come if we do not change the way we interact with the rest of nature. If we continue to disrupt and devastate the physical environment, it will simply bite back in the form of new diseases and pandemics.

Humans have altered ecosystems since prehistory and we know from thousands of years' bitter experience that diseases will continue to emerge and recur. Because we did not know better, or did not see the links between how we live and what we suffer, we have learned to live with them and normalised them. But with new knowledge of how and why infectious diseases start, there is no reason to accept that seasonal flu will kill tens of thousands of old people a year, that malaria will kill hundreds of thousands or that intensive farming will see vast numbers of diseased fish or poultry.

The era of medicate, vaccinate and then try to eradicate is over. We know now that it is the conditions in which life exists that determine plant, animal and human health and that it is mostly in our own hands how life continues to evolve. Until recently humanity had little choice but to be passive in the face of pandemics. It is only when we understand what is causing them that we can cease to be the prisoners of our own blindness and determine both our own health and that of other species.

With luck and reflection, the coronavirus pandemic may be seen to lead to a deeper understanding of the environmental ties that bind us together. Far from being helpless, we can avoid climate change and restore the nature of which we are a part, and therefore limit future infectious diseases. We may have created the conditions for them to emerge and spread but we also have the tools and the knowledge to change.

Only when we accept that we are responsible for most of the major diseases of the past few decades will we have the motivation to address them at source. Covid-19, Ebola, MERS, bird flu, HIV/ Aids and all the other pandemics we see cry out for us to change our relationship with the rest of nature.

ACKNOWLEDGEMENTS

This book was born and brought up in the Covid-19 lockdown when libraries were closed or inaccessible, travel was impossible and personal contacts limited. So it is with immense gratitude that I recognise the many people who inspired it and helped it and me through those unusual times.

I was lucky that Mary Hoff and David Doody at the University of Minnesota's Institute of the Environment sparked the idea and commissioned a piece for Ensia, David Godwin, London agent extraordinary, saw its potential to grow into a book and Jasmine Horsey at Bloomsbury had the courage and skill to run with it. Thanks also to Elisabeth Denison, Martha Jay and Richard Collins at Bloomsbury, who grappled with my typing and steered the book home.

Some chapters have drawn on pieces first published in the *Guardian* and *Observer*, so thanks to editors Alan Rusbridger, Kath Viner and Paul Webster, who for years licensed me to wander the world like some migratory bird.

Huge thanks are due, too, to the *Guardian*'s multi-disciplined environment, science, health and development desks. Damian Carrington, Adam Vaughan, Fiona Harvey, Ian Sample, Jonathan Watts, Patrick Barkham, Robin McKie, Bibi van der Zee, Karen McVeigh, Lucy Lamble, Eric Hilaire, Max Benato, Tom Levitt, Alan Evans, Karl Mathiesen and health editor Sarah Boseley have all been great colleagues, delightful to work with and kind enough to overlook my ignorance, share their experiences and put up with my long absences.

This book took me down many boulder-strewn journalistic paths that I had not followed before. Health and environment, science and culture, politics and social justice are often artificially separated so thanks to the many professors, researchers, veterinarians, historians, ecologists, conservationists and human rights and poverty workers in many countries who helped explain their work so well and join the dots. Richard Horton at the *Lancet* and Fiona Godley at the *British Medical Journal* gave me access to their databases, and, with Dr Robin Stott, former dean at Lewisham Hospital in London, who has done so much to put climate on the medical map, inspired me to think far more broadly about the links between health, poverty and nature; Thomas Gillespie at Emory, Felicia Keesing at Bard College and Rick Ostfeld at the Cary Institute were important, as were Chris Given-Wilson at St Andrews and Kate Jones at University College London. Thanks, too, to *Guardian* country diarist and wise ecologist Paul Evans for spelling out the links between human, animal and plant health.

Thanks, also, to GPs Rob Smith and Bill Seward in Wales, and for reading drafts and encouragement David Briant, Julia Armstrong, Sara Harker, Tony Meadows, Ferelith Smith, John and Pauline Smout, Alex Lewis, Allegra Vidal, Di Sherlock, Patience Foster, Peter North and Paul Manias.

'Queenie' Arekpitan in Lagos braved the bushmeat markets and hunters of Benin City, Jess Marais researched personal health and Sue Horsler, Tracey Hunter and John Craddock all rescued me with admin and IT skills. Thanks, too, to Delwyn and Teresa Northall and others on the Welsh border who kept me more or less sane as we huddled round braziers during lockdown.

But above all, my deep love and sincere thanks goes to Jen Bates, who, astonishingly and sometimes inexplicably, put up with me and kept me safe and laughing, and without whom this book would never have been possible.

NOTES

CHAPTER 1

1 Annals of Community Health, 'Emerging and Re-emerging Infectious Diseases', http://annalsofcommunityhealth.in, accessed 14 October 2022.

2 Steven Mithen, *After the Ice: A Global Human History, 20,000–5,000 BC*, Harvard University Press, Cambridge, MA, 2004, pp. 39–40.

3 Ethne Barnes, *Diseases and Human Evolution*, University of New Mexico Press, Albuquerque, 2007, pp. 10–11.

4 Mithen, *After the Ice*, p. 43.

5 Jack Harlan, *Crops and Man*, Crop Science Society of America, Madison, WI, 1992, p. 25.

6 C. A. Roberts and M. Cox, *Health and Disease in Britain: From Prehistory to the Present Day*, Alan Sutton Publishing, Gloucester, 2003.

7 Melissa Graboyes at https://africa.uoregon.edu/profile/graboyes, accessed 14 October 2022.

8 Melissa Graboyes, *The Experiment Must Continue: Medical Research and Ethics in East Africa, 1940–2014* (Perspectives on Global Health), Ohio University Press, Athens, OH, 2015, p. 18.

9 Andrew P. Dobson and E. Robin Carper, 'Infectious diseases and human population history: throughout history the establishment of disease has been a side effect of the growth of civilization', *Bioscience*, 46/2 (February 1996), https://academic.oup.com.

10 Barnes, *Diseases and Human Evolution*, p. 9.

11 Jared Diamond, 'The Worst Mistake in Human History', *Discover* (May 1987), pp. 64–6, https://web.cs.ucdavis.edu.

12 John Reader, *Cities*, William Heinemann, London, 2004, p. 16.

13 Ibid., p. 29.

14 Gwendolyn Leick, *Mesopotamia: The Invention of the City*, Penguin, Harmondsworth, 2003, p. 78.

15 Steven Mithen, interview with the author, 2021.

16 Ibid.

17 Donald R. Hopkins, *The Greatest Killer: Smallpox in History*, University of Chicago Press, Chicago, 2002.

18 At https://bible.knowing-jesus.com/topics/Plagues, accessed 18 October 2022.

19 Barnes, *Diseases and Human Evolution*, p. 51.

20 Reader, *Cities*, pp. 7–8.

21 Thucydides, *The Peloponnesian War*, 2.49.2–3, trans. Roger Crawley, at www.livius.org.

22 'Malaria', *International Encyclopaedia of the Social and Behavioural Sciences*, ed. Neil J. Smelser and Paul B. Baltes, Elsevier, Amsterdam, 2001.

23 Juan Peset, 'Plagues and Diseases in History', www.sciencedirect.com, accessed 18 October 2022.

24 Adomnán, Abbot of Iona, *De Locis Sanctis*, *c.* 680, www.birmingham.ac.uk/Documents/college-artslaw.

25 S. Sabbatani and S. Fiorino, 'The Antonine Plague and Decline of Rome' (in Italian), *Infezmed*, 17/4 (December 2009), pp. 261–75, https://pubmed.ncbi.nlm.nih.gov/20046111.

26 W. J. McLennan, 'The Eleven Plagues of Edinburgh', *Proceedings of the Royal College of Physicians, Edinburgh*, 31 (2001), pp. 256–61, www.rcpe.ac.uk.

27 'The Log of Christopher Columbus 1492', www.everything2.com, accessed 14 October 2022.

28 Noble David Cook, *Born to Die: Disease and New World Conquest*, Cambridge University Press, Cambridge, 1998, p. 48.

29 'Columbus' Second Voyage, 1493', https://usuaris.tinet.cat/evl/en/resumen2.htm, accessed 14 October 2022.

30 'The Black Death, Horseman of the Apocalypse in the Fourteenth Century', Missouri University, https://academic.mu.edu, accessed 14 October 2022.

31 M. Livi-Bacci, 'The Depopulation of Hispanic America after the Conquest', *Population and Development Review*, 32/2 (June 2006), pp. 199–232.

32 Roger G. Kennedy, *Mr. Jefferson's Lost Cause*, Oxford University Press, Oxford, 2004.

CHAPTER 2

1 CDC, 'Deaths Associated with Hurricane Georges', Morbidity Report, 1998.

2 P. Ranganathan and N. Raja, 'Reverse Zoonosis: When Humans Pass Disease on to Animals', www.science.thewire.in, 26 June 2020.

3 Bill Hathaway, 'Mass Animal Die Offs', https://news.yale.edu, 12 January 2015.

4 Kate Jones et al., 'Global Trends in Emerging Infectious Diseases', *Nature*, 451 (2008), www.nature.com.

5 Shahid Jarned et al., 'Global Biological Trends', *Journal Indian Institute of Science*, 100 (2020), https://link.springer.com.

6 K. F. Smith et al., 'Global Rise in Human Infectious Diseases', *Journal of the Royal Society, Interface*, 11/101 (2014), https://europe pmc.org.

7 Ibid.

8 World Economic Forum, 'Outbreak Readiness Impacts', http://outbreaks.globalincidentmap.com, accessed 14 October 2022.

9 Interview with the author, 2021.

10 Jeet Singh, 'Degradation of Biodiversity and Emergence of Zoonotic Diseases', https://health.ri.gov/diseases/infectious, 2020.

11 Melissa Kaplan, 'Symptom List of Lyme Disease', at www.anapsid.org, accessed 14 October 2022.

12 WHO, 'In Africa, 63% jump in diseases spread from animals to people seen in last decade', www.afro.who.int, 14 July 2022.

13 John Vidal, 'Zika forest, birthplace of a virus', www.theguardian.com, 13 February 2016.

14 Peter Daszak et al., 'A New Agenda for Emerging Diseases', https://doi.org/10.1196/annals.1307.001.

15 Gretchen C. Daily and Paul R. Ehrlich, 'Global Change and Human Susceptibility to Disease', *Annu. Rev. Energy Environ.*, 21 (1996), https://mahb.stanford.edu.

CHAPTER 3

1 Mike Collis, 'The Enslavement of Amazonian Natives During the Rubber Boom', www.iquitostimes.com, accessed 14 October 2022.

2 Wisconsin University, 'Major study links malaria mosquitos to deforestation', https://news.wisc.edu, 25 June 2009.

3 Amy Vittor et al., 'Epidemiology of Emerging Madariaga', *PloS Neglected Tropical Diseases*, 21 April 2016, https://journals.plos.org.

4 Amy Vittor et al., 'How Deforestation Helps Deadly Viruses Jump from Animals to Humans'. Phys.org 2020. https://phys.org/news/2020-06-deforestation-deadly-viruses-animals-humans.html.

5 Interview with the author, 2021.

6 Interview with the author, 2009.

7 Notice, Emergencia Indigena APIB, https://apiboficial.org, accessed 14 October 2022.

8 NBC News, 'Survival of Brazil's Indigenous groups hinges on urgent Covid response', www.nbc.com, 12 March 2021.

9 Ahssanuddin Haseeb, 'Why Zoonotic Diseases Are Fast Spreading in India', *Hyderabad News*, 2018, www.hydnews.net.

10 Nithyanand Rao, 'The Seven Decade Hunt for the Origins of Kyasanur Disease', https://science.thewire.in, 19 November 2016; Andrew J. MacDonald and Erin A. Mordecai, 'Amazon deforestation drives malaria transmission, and malaria burden reduces forest clearing', www.pnas.org, 14 October 2019.

11 Syed Shah et al., 'Epidemiology, pathogenesis, and control of a tick-borne disease: kyasanur forest disease: current status and future directions', *Front. Cell. Infect. Microbiol.*, 9 (May 2018), at www.frontiersin.org.

12 M. Sucitra, 'Jungle Virus Causes Concern', *Millennium Post*, 8 January 2015, at www.millenniumpost.in.

13 Interview with Kate Jones, 2021.

14 MacDonald and Mordecai, 'Amazon deforestation drives malaria transmission'.

15 Cirad, 'Covid-19: The Environmental Origin of the Pandemic', www.cirad.fr, 27 April 2020.

16 Montira Pongsiri et al., 'Biodiversity Affects Global Disease Ecology', *BioScience*, 59/11 (2009), https://academic.oup.com.

CHAPTER 4

1 Nasa, 'Smoke from Siberian Wildfires', https://modis.gsfc.nasa.gov, 7 August 2021.

2 Nasa Earth Observatory, 20 August 2021, 'Fires in Brazil, Paraguay, Argentina', https://earthobservatory.nasa.gov/images/11924/fires-in-brazil-argentina-and-paraguay

3 Agence France Presse, 'Smoke from Siberian wildfires reaches North Pole in historic first', www.theguardian.com, 9 August 2021.

4 Volker Radeloff et al., 'Rapid Growth of the US Wildland–Urban Interface Raises Wildfire Risk', *PNAS*, 115/13 (12 March 2018), www.pnas.org.

5 Yanis Varoufakis, 'Greece's wildfires', www.theguardian.com, 29 August 2021.

6 Ibid.

7 'Wildfires Increasing in Size and Frequency across Victoria', www.sciencedaily.com, 18 May 2020.

8 Associated Press, 'Lake Tahoe Threatened by Fire, More Ordered to Flee', www.thestar.com, 30 August 2021.

9 Genevieve Rajewski, 'The Consequences of Spraying Fire Retardants on Wildfires', Tufts Now, https://now.tufts.edu, 11 September 2020.

10 Fay Johnston et al., 'Estimate of Mortality Attributable to Smoke from Landscape Fires', *Environmental Health Perspectives*, 120/5 (1 May 2012), at https://ehp.niehs.nih.gov.

11 Hanno Seebens et al., 'No Saturation in the Accumulation of Alien Species Worldwide', *Nature Comms.*, 8 (15 February 2017), at www.nature.com.

12 CSIRO, 'Fighting Nipah Virus', www.csiro.au, accessed 14 October 2022.

13 Chua Kow Bing, 'Personal Account of Discovery of Nipah Virus', https://sites.google.com/site/class1979/nipah, accessed 14 October 2022.

14 Ibid.

15 Sohayati Rahman et al., 'Characterization of Nipah Virus from Naturally Infected *Pteropus vampyrus* Bats, Malaysia', *Emerging Infectious Diseases*, 16/12 (2010), at www.ncbi.nlm.nih.gov.

16 Ann Jeanette Glauber, 2016, 'Seeing the Impact of Forest Fires, https://blogs.worldbank.org/voices/seeing-impact-forest-fires-south-sumatra-view-field

17 Interview with Yuyun Indradi, Jakarta 2015.

18 Shannon N. Koplitz et al., 'Public Health Impacts of the Severe Haze in Equatorial Asia in September–October 2015: Demonstration of a New Framework for Informing Fire Management Strategies to Reduce Downwind Smoke Exposure', Environmental Research Letters, http://iopscience.iop.org, 19 September 2016.

19 V. Huijnen et al., 2016 'Fire Carbon Emissions Over SE Asia 2015, https://www.cifor.org/publications/pdf_files/articles/AGaveau1603.pdf

20 Center for International Forestry Research, 'Life Amid the Fires and Haze of Central Kalimantan', https://forestsnews.cifor.org, 27 October 2015.

21 World Bank, Report, 'Cost of Fires in Indonesia', at https://documents.worldbank.org/en/publication/documents-reports/documentdetail/776101467990969768/the-cost-of-fire-an-economic-analysis-of-indonesia-s-2015-fire-crisis

22 Seema Jayachandran, 'Air Quality and Early-Life Mortality: Evidence from Indonesia's Wildfires', Journal of Human Resources, 44/4 (Fall 2009), at www.jstor.org.

23 Ibid.

CHAPTER 5

1 Interviews with the author, Aralsk, Kazakhstan 2012.

2 Ibid.

3 Ibid.

4 Ibid.

5 Nick Middleton, Extremes Along the Silk Road, John Murray, London, 2005.

6 Nick Middleton, Going to Extremes: Voz-Island (Vozrozhdeniya) – Part 1, www.youtube.com, 2 April 2008.

7 Middleton, Extremes Along the Silk Road.

8 Interview Stephan Mantel, 2021.

9 IPBES, 'Report on Land Degradation and Restoration', https://ipbes.net, accessed 14 October 2022.

10 Evan Thaler et al., 'The Extent of Soil Loss across the US Corn Belt', *PNAS*, 118/8 (2020), at www.pnas.org.

11 UN Convention to Combat Desertification, 'Global Land Outlook 2017', www.unccd.int, accessed 14 October 2022.

12 Lynn Peeples, 'Dust Storms' Health Risks: Asthma Triggers, Chemicals, Bacteria May Be in the Wind', www.huffingtonpost. co.uk, 11 August 2012.

13 Kansas Historical Society, 'Dust Bowl 1931', at www.kshs.org, accessed 14 October 2022.

14 Timothy Egan, *The Worst Hard Time: The Untold Story of Those Who Survived the Great American Dust Bowl*, Mariner Books, Boston, 2006; Sam Heft-Neal et al., 'Dust pollution from the Sahara and African infant mortality', *Nature Sustainability*, 3 (2020), www.nature.com.

15 Daniel Tong, 'Intensified Dust Storm Activity and Valley Fever Infection in the Southwestern United States', *Geophysical Research Letters*, 44/9 (2017), at https://agupubs.onlinelibrary.wiley.com.

16 Nick Middleton, 'Dust Storm Hazards', at www.researchgate.net, January 2019.

17 Hugh Bronstein, 'Analysis: Lack of crop rotation slowly turns Argentine Pampas into "sand"', www.reuters.com, 23 October 2013.

18 Liu et al., 'Changing Climate and Overgrazing are Decimating Mongolian Steppes' 2013, *PlosOne*, 8, 57599. 1–6, doi; 10.1371/journal. pone 0057599

19 Y. Chen and H. Tang, 'Desertification in North China: background, anthropogenic impacts and failures in combating it', *Land Degradation and Development*, 16 (2005), www.igsnrr.cas.cn.

20 Jorqura Hector et al., 'Association of Kawasaki disease with tropospheric winds in Central Chile: is wind-borne desert dust a risk factor?', *Environ Int.* (May 2015), at https://pubmed.ncbi.nlm.nih.gov.

21 Nick Middleton, 'Dust Storm Hazards', at www.researchgate.net, January 2019.

22 Rachel Cernansky, 'Taking root: A new influx of funds could help realize Africa's Great Green Wall', *Science Magazine*, February 2021, at www.sciencemag.org.

23 Ziad Memish et al, *Lancet*, 2019, 'Mass Gatherings Medicine; Public Health Issues arising from Religious and Sporting events', https://www.thelancet.com/journals/lancet/article/PIIS0 140-6736%2814%2960851-5/fulltext

24 Chen and Tang, 'Desertification in North China'.

25 S. Perkins-Kirkpatrick and S. C. Lewis, 'Increasing trends in regional heatwaves', *Nature Comms.*, 11 (2020), at www.nature.com.

26 Interview with Patricio Garcia-Fayos, 2005.

27 UNDP, 'Sudan National Adaptation Programme of Action (NAPA)', www.adaptation-undp.org, accessed 15 October 2022.

28 Wang Tao, *Desertification in Western China*, Taylor & Francis, London, 1998.

29 FAO, 'Soil Pollution Jeopardising Life on Earth', https://news.un.org, December 2018.

30 FAO, 'Global Assessment of Soil Pollution', www.fao.org, accessed 15 October 2022.

31 Damian Carrington, 'World's soils "under great pressure", says UN pollution report', www.theguardian.com, 4 June 2011.

CHAPTER 6

1 Alfred Newton, 'Abstract of Mr J. Wolley's Researches in Iceland Regarding the Great Auk', 1861, at https://onlinelibrary.wiley.com.

2 Ibid.

3 Interview with Bob Watson, 2018.

4 Elizabeth Hadly, interviewed in *Extinction: The Facts*, BBC One, 13 September 2020.

5 Kathy Willis, interviewed in *Extinction: The Facts*, BBC One, 13 September 2020.

6 Juliette Jowit, 'Humans driving extinction faster than species can evolve, say experts', www.theguardian.com, 7 March 2010.

7 Ibid.

8 Shi-Lin Chen et al., 'Conservation and sustainable use of medicinal plants: problems, progress, and prospects', *Chin Med.* (July 2016), www.ncbi.nlm.nih.gov.

9 Susan Mayor, 'Tree that provides Paclitaxel is put on list of endangered species', *British Medical Journal* (November 2011), www.bmj.com.

10 'Artemisia annual', at https://en.wikipedia.org, accessed 15 October 2022.

11 Save the Amazon Coalition, www.savetheamazon.org/rainforeststats.htm

12 ETC Group, 'Report on Bioprospecting and Biopiracy', 1996, at www.etcgroup.org.

13 Jamie Johnson, 'Florida prepares to release 750m GM mosquitoes', www.telegraph.co.uk, 27 April 2021.

14 Jane Dalton, 'Exterminating bats blamed for spreading Covid-19 would increase risk of further diseases, warn experts', www.independ ent.co.uk, 24 April 2020.

15 Elizabeth Hadly, Stanford University profile, https://news.stanford. edu, 30 March 2021.

16 Fiona Harvey, 'Bison recovering but 31 other species now extinct, says red list', www.theguardian.com, 10 December 2020.

17 Interview with Christine Kreuder Johnson, 2021.

18 F. Keesing et al., 'Effect of Species Diversity on Disease Risk', *Ecology Letters* (March 2006), https://onlinelibrary.wiley.com.

19 Interviews with Rick Ostfeld, Felicia Keesing, 2021, 2022.

20 Ibid.

21 Ibid.

22 International Livestock Research institute (ILRI), 'Preventing the next pandemic: zoonotic diseases and how to break the chain of transmission', www.ilri.org, 6 July 2020.

CHAPTER 7

1 Lydia Morris, 'Lyme Disease on Rise in Wales', www.dailypost.co.uk, 2 July 2018.

2 D. Sprenger and T. Wulthiranyagool, 'The discovery and distribution of *Aedes albopictus* in Harris County, Texas', American Mosquito Control Association, https://pubmed.ncbi.nlm.nih.gov/3507493, 1986/

3 European Centre for Disease Prevention, '*Aedes albopictus* Current Known Distribution March 2021', www.ecdc.europa.eu, 31 March 2021.

4 Interview with Michael Weissman, 2021.

5 Interview with Elena Tricarico, 2021.

6 Interview with Nagat El Tayeb, 2009.

7 Interview with Bukar Tijani, 2010.

8 Interview with Moqbal Hossain, 2013.

9 Hanna Seebens et al., 'No saturation in the accumulation of alien species worldwide', *Nature Comms.*, www.nature.com, 15 February 2017.

10 M. Kirchmair et al., 'Biological control of Grape Phylloxera: a historical review and future prospects', *Acta Hortic.*, 816 (2009), www. actahort.org.

11 'The American Plagues', www.vinetowinecircle.com, accessed 18 October 2022; David Steadman, 'Bird populations and species lost to Late Quaternary environmental change and human impact in the Bahamas', *PNAS*, 117 (5 October 2020), www.pnas.org.

12 Morgane Barbet-Massin et al., 'The economic cost of control of the invasive yellow-legged Asian hornet', *NeoBiota*, 55 (3 April 2020), https://DOI:10.3897/neobiota.55.38550.

13 Tim Blackburn et al., 'Alien species are the primary cause of global extinctions', www.ucl.ac.uk, 4 April 2019.

14 '10 invasive species threatening Canadian habitats', www.cbc.ca, 27 February 2012.

15 David Pimentel et al., 'Update on the environmental and economic costs associated with alien-invasive species in the United States', *Ecological Economics*, 52, www.sciencedirect.com, 15 February 2005.

16 Stephanie Pain, 'Why Tree-Killing Epidemics are on the Rise', www. smithsonianmag.com, 28 September 2020.

17 Seebens et al., 'No saturation'.

CHAPTER 8

1 Interview with Arne Sorensen, 2012.

2 Ibid.

3 Interview with Nick Toberg, 2012.

4 Ed Struzik, 'Is Warming Bringing a Wave of New Diseases to Arctic Wildlife?', https://e360.yale.edu, 6 November 2018.

5 Greg Allen, 'Florida Citrus Near a Comeback', NPR Radio, www. npr.org, 4 December 2016.

6 Interview with Daniel Brooks, 2022.

7 Ibid.

8 Ibid.

9 Colin Carlson et al., 'Climate change increases cross-species viral transmission risk', *Nature*, 607, www.nature.com, 28 April 2022.

10 Timothee Poisot, Twitter April 2022, https://twitter.com/tpoi/status/1519677023786090496

11 Asim Anwal et al., 'Climate Change and Infectious Diseases: Evidence from Highly Vulnerable Countries', *Iranian Journal of Public Health*, 48/12 (December 2019), www.ncbi.nlm.nih.gov.

12 Monroe County, Florida official website, at www.monroecounty-fl. gov, accessed 17 October 2022.

13 Ibid.

14 Interview with Mark Whitside, 2020.

15 Ibid.

16 Michael X. Tong et al., 'Dengue control in the context of climate change: Views from health professionals in different geographic regions of China', *Journal of Infection and Public Health*, 12/3 (May 2019), www.sciencedirect.com.

17 James Messina and Oliver Brody, 'A New Picture of Dengue's Growing Threat', www.geog.ox.ac.uk, 24 June 2019.

18 Xiaoxu Wu et al., 'Impact of climate change on human infectious diseases: Empirical evidence and human adaptation', *Environment International*, 86 (January 2016), www.sciencedirect.com.

19 Interview with PAGASA, 2014.

20 Interview with Denis Posada, 2014.

21 Interview with Yeb Sano, 2014.

22 O. F. Wilhelmi et al., 'Compounding hazards and intersecting vulnerabilities: experiences and responses to extreme heat during COVID-19', *Env. Letters*, 16/8 (6 August 2021), https://iopscience. iop.org.

23 Cascade Tuholske et al., 'Global urban population exposure to extreme heat', *PNAS*, 118/41 (3 December 2020), www.pnas.org.

24 Colin Raymond et al., 'The emergence of heat and humidity too severe for human tolerance', *Science Advances*, 6/19 (8 May 2020), www.science.org.

25 Jeff Asher, 'A Rise in Murder? Let's Talk About the Weather', www. nytimes.com, 21 September 2019.

26 Shakoor Hajat et al., 'Climate change effects on human health: projections of temperature-related mortality for the UK during the 2020s, 2050s and 2080s', *Journal of Epidemiology and Human Health*, 68/7 (2014), https://jech.bmj.com.

27 Raymond et al., 'The emergence of heat'; NOAA, 'Dangerous humid heat extremes occurring decades before expected', https://research. noaa.gov, 8 May 2020.

28 NOAA, 'Dangerous humid heat extremes'.

29 Jonas Jagermeyer, 'Global Climate Change Impact on Crops Expected Within 10 Years, NASA Study Finds', www.nasa.gov, 1 November 2021.

30 UN News, 'Heatwave to Affect Almost Every Child on Earth by 2050', https://news.un.org/en/story/2022/10/1129852

31 FAO, 'State of Food Security 2021', www.fao.org, accessed 18 October 2022.

32 Interview with Pensulo Phiri, 2015.

33 Marco Springmann et al., 'Global and health effects of future food production under climate change: a modelling study', *The Lancet*, 387/10021 (7 May 2016), www.thelancet.com.

34 Stephane Hallegatte et al., *Shock Waves: Managing the Impacts of Climate Change on Poverty*, https://openknowledge.worldbank.org.

35 '2019 Lancet Coundown on Health and Climate Change: Policy Brief for the U.S.', www.hsph.harvard.edu, 13 November 2022.

36 Sharanjit Leyl, 'Mark Carney: Climate crisis deaths will be "worse than Covid"', www.bbc.co.uk, 5 February 2021.

CHAPTER 9

1 Lancelot Hogben, 'History of the Hogben Test', *British Medical Journal* (October 1946), www.bmj.com.

2 Dan Greenberg and Wendy Palen, 'A Deadly Amphibian Disease Goes Global', *Science*, 2019, https://www.science.org/doi/10.1126/science.aax0002

3 Bruno Chomel et al., 'Wildlife, Exotic Pets, and Emerging Diseases', *Emerging Infectious Diseases*, 13/1 (January 2017), wwwnc.cdc.gov/eid/article/13/1/06-0480_article.

4 G. T. Keusch et al., *Drivers of Zoonotic Disease*, National Academies Press, Washington, DC, 2009, www.ncbi.nlm.nih.gov/books/NBK215318; Tiffany A. Yap et al., 'Averting a North American biodiversity crisis', *Science*, 349/6247 (July 2015), www.researchgate.net; World Animal Protection, 'UK Imports Wild Animals from Known Disease Hotspots', www.worldanimalprotection.org.uk, 21 September 2020.

5 William Karesh et al., 'Wildlife Trade and Global Disease Emergence', *Emerging Infectious Diseases*, 11/7 (July 2005), www.ncbi.nlm.nih.gov.

6 'Global wildlife trade a key factor in species decline', www.ft.com, 3 October 2019.

7   'HIV and Aids: An Origin Story', www.publichealth.org, accessed 18 October 2022.

8   Diana Bell et al., 'Animal origins of SARS coronavirus: possible links with the international trade in small carnivores', *Philos. Trans. R. Soc. Lond. B. Biol. Sci.*, 359/1447 (July 2004), www.ncbi.nlm.nih.gov.

9   Steven van Borm et al., 'Highly pathogenic H5N1 virus in smuggled Thai eagles, Belgium', *Emerg. Infect. Dis.*, 11/5 (May 2005), www.ncbi.nlm.nih.gov.

10 Victor Siamudaaia, 'A study of the epidemiology and socio-economic impact of anthrax in Luangwa Valley in Zambia', https://repository.up.ac.za, 9 March 2006.

11 Larisa Lee-Cruz et al., 'Mapping of Ebola virus spillover: Suitability and seasonal variability at the landscape scale', *PloS Neglected Tropical Diseases*, www.researchgate.net, 23 August 2001.

12 Julia Fa et al., 'Bushmeat exploitation in tropical forests: an intercontinenal comparison'. *Conservation Biology*, 16/1 (2002), www.researchgate.net.

13 Theodore Trefon,'Bushmeat: the culture and economy of eating wild animals in Central Africa', www.africamuseum.be, 20 February 2020.

14 Interview with the author.

15 Ibid.

16 Joe Pinkstone, 'Inside Africa's Wet Markets', www.dailymail.co.uk, 19 February 2021.

17 Interview with Thomas Gillespie, 2022.

18 Jesse Bonwitt et al., 'Unintended Consequences of the "Bushmeat ban" in West Africa during the 2013–2016 Ebola virus disease epidemic', *Social Science and Medicine*, 200 (March 2018), www.sciencedirect.com.

19 Interview with 'Queenie' Arekpitan at Oluwo Market, 2020.

20 Eric Fèvre and Cecilia Tacoli, 'Coronavirus threat looms large for low income cities', www.iied.org, 26 February 2020.

21 Mama Mouamfon and Cedric Tagne, 'How is Covid-19 affecting wild meat consumption in Cameroon?', www.iied.org, 20 November 2020.

22 B. Lee Lignon, 'Monkeypox: A review of the history and emergence in the Western hemisphere', *Seminars in Pediatric Infectious Diseases*, 15/4 (October 2004), www.sciencedirect.com.

23 Centres for Disease Control, 'Monkeypox Past Cases', www.cdc.gov, accessed 18 October 2022.

24 'Census Bureau Statistics on Pets', www.census.gov, 7 April 2017.

25 Centres for Disease Control, 'Diseases That Can Spread between Animals and People', www.cdc.gov, accessed 18 October 2022.

26 Interview with Bruno Chomel, 2021.

27 Ibid.

28 Ioannis Magouras et al., 'Emerging zoonotic diseases: should we rethink the animal–human interface?', *Sec. Veterinary Epidemiology and Economics* (22 October 2020), www.frontiersin.org.

29 FAO, 'Wildlife Farming in Viet Nam', www.fao.org, accessed 18 October 2022.

30 Michaeleen Doucleff, 'WHO Points to Wildlife Farms in China as Likely Source of Pandemic', www.npr.org, 15 March 2021.

31 Ibid.

32 See Julia Fa et al., 'Mapping the availability of Bushmeat for consumption in Central African cities', *Environmental Research Letters*, 14 (2019), https://iopscience.iop.org.

CHAPTER 10

1 Walter Plowright, 'Presentation of the 1999 World Food Prize Laureate', www.fao.org, accessed 19 October 2022.

2 Peter Roeder, 'Rinderpest: the end of cattle plague', *Preventive Veterinary Medicine*, 102/2 (2011), www.sciencedirect.com.

3 Interview with Richard Pankhurst, 2012.

4 David M. Morens et al., 'Global Rinderpest Eradication: Lessons Learned and Why Humans should Celebrate Too', *Journal of Infectious Diseases*, 204/4 (2011), https://academic.oup.com.

5 T. Barrett and P. Rossiter, 'Rinderpest: the disease and its impact on humans and animals', *Adv. Virus Research*, 53 (1999), https://pubmed.ncbi.nlm.nih.gov.

6 Begna F. Duggasa, 'Colonialism and Public Health: The Case of the Rinderpest Virus in Oromia Regional State in Ethiopia', *Journal of Preventive Medicine* (January 2018), https://preventive-medicine.imedpub.com.

7 Fred Pearce, 'Why Africa's National Parks are Failing to Save Wildlife', https://e360.yale.edu, 19 January 2020.

8 Simon Willis, '1843 travel map', *The Economist*, www.economist.com, 23 September 2019.

9 J. N. Hays, 'Seventh Cholera Pandemic', https://en.wikipedia.org, accessed 19 October 2022.

10 Ethne Barnes, *Diseases and Human Evolution*, University of New Mexico Press, Albuquerque, 2005, p. 285.

11 'On Sea-Borne Cholera: British Measures of Prevention v. European Measures of Restriction', *British Medical Journal* (13 August 1887), www.bmj.com.

12 Jack Chadwick, 'The Cholera Riots', https://tribunemag.co.uk, July 2020.

13 Mihaela Oprea et al., 'The seventh pandemic of cholera in Europe revisited by microbial genomics', *Nature Comms.*, 11 (2020), www.nature.com.

14 S. McCarthy and F. Khambaty, 'International dissemination of epidemic Vibrio cholerae by cargo ship ballast and other non potable waters', *Applied. Environ. Microbiology*, 60/7 (1996), www.ncbi.nlm.nih.gov.

15 Charmain Ng et al., 'Occurrence of *Vibrio* species, beta-lactam resistant *Vibrio* species, and indicator bacteria in ballast and port waters of a tropical harbour', *Science of the Total Environment*, 610–11 (January 2018), www.sciencedirect.com.

16 Dana Wusinich-Mendez, 'Ballast Water Driving Coral Disease', University of South Florida radio, https://wusfnews.wusf.usf.edu, 4 February 2020.

17 Thomas Gale Moore, 'Protection in the Age of Cholera', https://web.stanford.edu, accessed 19 October 2022.

18 McCarthy and Khambaty, 'Dissemination of Cholera by Cargo Ship Ballast'.

19 'Summary of Confirmed Cases', https://en.wikipedia.org, accessed 19 October 2022.

20 Ontario Blue Cross, 'Contagious Diseases on Cruise Ships', https://qc.bluecross.ca, 1 September 2014.

21 Kara Tardivel et al., 'Travel by Air, Land and Sea', wwwnc.cdc.gov, accessed 19 October 2022.

22 Adele Marshall, 'Ship's log of the *USS Leviathan* 1919', https://archive.org, accessed 19 October 2022.

23 Ibid.

24 Serge Morand and Bruno Walther, 'The accelerated infectious disease risk in the Anthropocene: more outbreaks and wider global spread', www.biorxiv.org, 20 April 2020.

25 Ibid.

26 Katherine F. Smith et al., 'Global rise in human infectious disease outbreaks', *Journal of the Royal Society Interface*, 11/101 (December 2014), https://royalsocietypublishing.org.

27 Morand and Walther, 'Accelerated infectious disease risk in the Anthropocene'.

28 World Bank, 'Global Air Passenger Numbers', https://data.worldbank.org, accessed 19 October 2022.

29 Ellen Nakashima, 'Sars Signals Missed in Hong Kong', *Washington Post*, www.washingtonpost.com, 20 May 2003.

30 Interview with Jamie Bartram, 2020.

31 M. E. Wilson, 1995. Travel and the Emergence of Infectious Diseases. Emerging Infectious Diseases. DOI: 10.3201/eid0102.950201.

CHAPTER 11

1   Statista, 'Number of Chickens Worldwide from 1990 to 2020', www.statista.com, accessed 19 October 2022.

2   'Flu Deaths', https://usafacts.org, accessed 19 October 2022.

3   WHO, 'Seasonal Influenza fact sheet', www.who.int, accessed 19 October 2022.

4   US Department of Agriculture, 'New analysis shows overall increase in global poultry production, but with Europe lagging', www.thepoultrysite.com, 15 October 2021.

5   Leen Vijgen et al., 'Complete Genomic Sequence of Human Coronavirus OC43: Molecular Clock Analysis Suggests a Relatively Recent Zoonotic Coronavirus Transmission Event', *Journal of Virology* (1 February 2005), https://journals.asm.org.

6   Harald Brüssow, 'What we can learn from the dynamics of the 1889 "Russian flu" pandemic for the future trajectory of COVID-19', *Microbial Biotechnology* (31 August 2021), https://sfamjournals.onlinelibrary.wiley.com.

7   Mark Osborne Humphries, 'Paths of Infection: The First World War and the Origins of the 1918 Influenza Pandemic', *War in History*, 21/1 (January 2014), www.jstor.org.

8 WW1 Centenary, 'The Etaples Flu Pandemic?', http://ww1centenary. oucs.ox.ac.uk, accessed 19 October 2022.

9 J. S. Oxford et al., 'A hypothesis: the conjunction of soldiers, gas, pigs, ducks, geese and horses in Northern France during the Great War provided the conditions for the emergence of the "Spanish" influenza pandemic of 1918–1919', *Vaccine*, 23/7 (4 January 2005), www.sciencedirect.com.

10 David Payne, 'The Influenza Pandemic of 1918', www.westernfront association.com, accessed 19 October 2022.

11 Ann H. Reid et al., 'Origin and evolution of the 1918 "Spanish" influenza virus hemagglutinin gene', *Biological Sciences*, 96/4 (1999), www.pnas.org.

12 Oxford et al., 'A hypothesis'.

13 Svenn-Erik Mamelund, 'In 1918 Flu Pandemic, Mortality in Urban and Isolated Rural Areas Varied', www.infectioncontroltoday.com, 27 April 2011.

14 Claire Jackson, 'History lessons: the Asian Flu pandemic', *Journal of General Practice*, 59/565 (2009), https://bjgp.org.

15 BBC Radio History Hour, 'The 1957 Pandemic', www.bbc.co.uk, 2 May 2020.

16 Mark Honigsbaum, 'Revisiting the 1957 and 1968 influenza pandemics', *The Lancet*, 395/10240 (13 June 2020), www.thelan cet.com.

17 L. D. Sims et al., 'Avian Influenza in Hong Kong 1997–2002', *Avian Diseases*, 47/3 (September 2003), https://bioone.org.

18 K. F. Shortridge et al., 'The next influenza pandemic: lessons from Hong Kong', *Journal of Applied Microbiology*, 94/1 (May 2003), https://sfamjournals.onlinelibrary.wiley.com.

19 Mike Davis, *The Monster at our Door: The Global Threat of Avian Flu*, New Press, New York, 2005, pp. 105–6.

20 Annie Underwood, 'Scary Strains', www.newsweek.com, 31 October 2004.

21 Shortridge et al., 'The next influenza pandemic'. René Snacken et al., 'The Next Influenza Pandemic: Lessons from Hong Kong, 1997', *Journal of Emerging Infectious Diseases*, 5/2 (April 1999), wwwnc. cdc.gov.

22 Sims et al., 'Avian Influenza in Hong Kong 1997–2002'.

23 Barack Obama and Richard Lugar, 'Grounding a Pandemic', www.nytimes.com, 6 June 2005.

24 Yoshihiro Kawaoka et al., 'Bird Flu Slow to Infect Humans', www.cidrap.umn.edu, March 2020.

25 WHO, 'Human infection with avian influenza A(H5) viruses', www.who.int, 1 April 2022.

CHAPTER 12

1 K. F. Shortridge, 'Influenza: a continuing detective story', *The Lancet*, 354/SIV29 (1 December 1999), www.thelancet.com.

2 Xinjian Yan, 'The changing face of the world of duck production', *International Hatchery Practice*, 18/6 (2018), www.positiveaction.info.

3 Kennedy Shortridge, 'Avian influenza: A viruses of southern China and Hong Kong: ecological aspects and implications for man', *Bulletin of the World Health Organization*, 60/1 (1982), https://apps.who.int.

4 Ibid.

5 Carl Heneghan and Tom Jefferson, 'Covid-19 Deaths Compared with "Swine Flu"',www.cebm.net, 9 April 2020.

6 Martha Nelson, 'The Hunt for a Pandemic's Origins', www.the-scientist.com, January 2022.

7 WHO, 'Avian Flu Infects Humans in Russian Federation', www.euro.who.int, March 2021.

8 'Data on H5N8 Isolated from Russian Poultry Worker', *Eurosurveillance*, 26/24 (17 June 2021), www.poultrymed.com.

9 Kim Woo-Hyun and Seongbeom Cho, 'Estimation of the Basic Reproduction Numbers of the Subtypes H5N1, H5N8, and H5N6 During the Highly Pathogenic Avian Influenza Epidemic Spread Between Farms', *Frontiers in Veterinary Science*, 8 (2021), www.ncbi.nlm.nih.gov.

10 Anna Smolchenko and Amelie Baubau, 'Russia Just Alerted the WHO to the World's First Case of H5N8 Avian Flu in Humans', www.sciencealert.com, 22 February 2021.

11 'Avian influenza in wild birds', www.gov.uk, 30 December 2016.

12 IISD/FwUNEP, 'Summary report, 10–11 April 2006: Scientific Seminar on Avian Influenza, the Environment and Migratory Birds', https://enb.iisd.org, 10–11 April 2006.

13 Bryony Jones et al., 'Zoonosis emergence linked to agricultural intensification and environmental change', *Proc. Natl. Sci. USA*, 21/110 (May 2013), www.ncbi.nlm.nih.gov.

14 Fiona Harvey et al., 'Rise of mega farms: how the US model of intensive farming is invading the world', www.theguardian.com, 18 July 2017.

15 FAO, 'Surge in diseases of animal origin necessitates new approach to health – report', www.fao.org, 16 December 2013.

16 Ibid.

17 FAO, 'World Livestock 2013: Changing disease landscapes', www. fao.org. 2013.

18 Interview with the author.

19 M. Zuidhof et al., 'Growth, efficiency, and yield of commercial broilers from 1957, 1978, and 2005', *Poultry Science*, 93/12 (2014), https://pubmed.ncbi.nlm.nih.gov.

20 Interview with the author.

21 M. Zuidhof et al., 'The broiler chicken as a signal of a human reconfigured biosphere', *Royal Society Open Science*, 5/12 (December 2018), www.researchgate.net.

22 Statista, 'Number of Chickens Worldwide'.

23 Zuidhof et al., 'The broiler chicken'.

24 Interview with Rob Wallace, 2022.

25 Marius Gilbert et al., 'Intensifying poultry production systems and the emergence of avian influenza in China: a "One Health/ Ecohealth" epitome', *Arch. Public Health*, 75/48 (November 2017), https://pubmed.ncbi.nlm.nih.go.

26 Ibid.

27 Madhur Dhingra et al., 'Geographical and Historical Patterns in the Emergences of Novel Highly Pathogenic Avian Influenza (HPAI) H5 and H7 Viruses in Poultry', *Frontiers in Veterinary Science*, 5 (June 2018), www.researchgate.net.

28 BBC Science Focus, 'Bacteria', www.sciencefocus.com, accessed 20 October 2022.

29 BBC Science Focus, 'Viruses', www.sciencefocus.com, accessed 20 October 2022.

30 'Intensive farming increases risk of epidemics', www.sciencedaily. com, 4 May 2020.

31 Ibid.; BBC Science Focus, 'Coronavirus', www.sciencefocus.com, accessed 20 October 2022.

32 'Intensive farming increases risk of epidemics', www.sciencedaily. com, 4 May 2020.

33 Ibid.

34 Interview with Samuel K. Sheppard, 2022.

35 Montserrat Agüero et al., 'Highly pathogenic avian influenza A(H5N1) virus infection in farmed minks, Spain, October 2022' in *Eurosurveillance* (Volume 28, Issue 3, 19/Jan/2023), https://www.eurosurveillance.org/content/10.2807/1560-7917. ES.2023.28.3.2300001.

CHAPTER 13

1 James Cowden and John Duffy, *The Elder Dempster Fleet History, 1852–1985*, Mallett & Bell, Norfolk, 1986, pp. 243–7.

2 Nidal A-Z Kram et al., '"Making the most of our situation": a qualitative study reporting health providers' perspectives on the challenges of implementing the prevention of mother-to-child transmission of HIV services in Lagos, Nigeria', *BMJ Open*, 11/10 (October 2021), https://bmjopen.bmj.com.

3 Economist Intelligence Unit, 'Global Livability Index 2021', www.ias abhiyan.com, accessed 20 October 2022.

4 Chikwe Ihekweazu, 'As Nigeria Battles Multiple Concurrent Disease Outbreaks', https://headtopics.com, July 2021.

5 Layi Ehgunjobi, 'Tackling Africa's Slums', https://apps.who.int/iris/ handle/10665/48539

6 Olukayode A. Faleye, 'Environmental Change, Sanitation and Bubonic Plague in Lagos, 1924–31', *International Review of Environmental History* (2017), www.academia.edu.

7 Ibid.

8 Interview with Layi Ehgunjobi, 2013.

9 Ehgunjobi, 'Tackling Africa's Slums', https://apps.who.int/iris/han dle/10665/48539

10 Mohammad Sorowar Hossain et al., 'Chikungunya outbreak (2017) in Bangladesh: Clinical profile, economic impact and quality of life during the acute phase of the disease', *PLoS Neglected Tropical Diseases*, https://journals.plos.org, 6 June 2018.

11 'Nine per cent of Dhaka Infected with Covid-19', https://bdnews24. com, 11 August 2020.

12 Priya Shetty, 'Health Care for Urban Poor Falls through the Gap', *The Lancet*, 277/9766 (February 2011), www.thelancet.com.

13 Ibid.

14 Interview with Sam Brody, 2019.

15 Abiodun O. Oluyomi et al., 'Houston hurricane Harvey health (Houston-3H) study: assessment of allergic symptoms and stress after hurricane Harvey flooding', *Environmental Health*, 20 (January 2021), https://ehjournal.biomedcentral.com.

16 M. K. Nidheesh, 'Seven reasons why Bengaluru is growing to become an unlivable city', www.livemint.com, 24 June 2016.

17 Interview with T. V. Ramachandra, 2019.

18 'Greenpeace Clean Air Report'. https://unearthed.greenpeace.org, 22 February 2016.

19 Interview with T. V. Ramachandra, 2019.

20 Adriana Kocornik-Mina et al., 'Flooded Cities', *American Journal of Applied Economics*, 12/2 (2015), https://pubs.aeaweb.org.

CHAPTER 14

1 Interview with Mark Woolhouse, 2022.

2 Daszak, 'We Knew Disease X Was Coming. It's Here Now', www. nytimes.com, 27 February 2020.

3 Interview with Tom Koch, 2020.

4 Interview with Paul Gallagher, the *i*, 2020. 'World could face another pandemic "within 5 to 8 years", https://inews.co.uk/news/health/world-face-another-pandemic-tom-koch-predicted-coronavi rus-460702.

5 World Economic Forum, 'This is how we prevent future pandemics, say 22 leading scientists', www.weforum.org, 27 November 2020.

6 David M. Morens and Anthony S. Fauci, 'Emerging Pandemic Diseases: How We Got to COVID-19', *Cell*, 184/5 (3 September 2020), www.sciencedirect.com.

7 David M. Morens and Joel Brenan, 'Coming to Terms with the Real Terrorist Behind Covid-19: Nature', www.statnews.com, 9 September 2020.

8   World Economic Forum, 'Scientists warn worse pandemics are on the way if we don't protect nature', www.weforum.org, 4 May 2020.

9   Romain Espinosa et al., 'Infectious Diseases and Meat Production', *Environ. Resour. Econ. (Dordr)*, 76/4 (2020), www.ncbi.nlm.nih.gov.

10 Serge Morand and Bruno Walther, 'The accelerated infectious disease risk in the Anthropocene: more outbreaks and wider global spread', www.biorxiv.org, 20 April 2020.

11 Ibid.

12 Ibid.

13 Lina Awada et al., 'Current Animal Health Situation Worldwide: Analysis of Events and Trends', World Assembly of the OIE, Paris, 24–28 May 2021, https://web.oie.int.

14 'Covid: First UK case in pet dog confirmed by top vet', www.bbc.co.uk, 11 November 2021.

15 Sandra Diaz et al., 'Summary for policymakers of the global assessment report on biodiversity and ecosystem services of the Intergovernmental Science-Policy Platform on Biodiversity and Ecosystem Services', https://ec.europa.eu, 6 May 2019.

16 G. Allard et al., 'Global information on outbreaks and impact of major forest insect pests and diseases', www.fao.org, 2003.

17 Ramya Dwivedi, 'Game Animals as Potential Drivers of Disease', www.news-medical.net, 17 November 2021.

18 'Military Spending by Country', https://en.wikipedia.org, accessed 20 October 2022.

19 WHO, 'Health Spending by Country', www.who.int, accessed 20 October 2022.

20 WHO, 'MERS global summary', https://apps.who.int, accessed 20 October 2022.

21 Alice N. Kiyong'a et al., 'Middle East Respiratory Syndrome Coronavirus (MERS-CoV) Seropositive Camel Handlers in Kenya', *Viruses*, 12/4 (2020), www.mdpi.com.

22 German Centre for Infection Research 'Promising MERS coronavirus vaccine trial in humans', www.sciencedaily.com, 22 April 2020.

23 Interview with Delia Grace Randolph, 2020.

24 M. Rozo and G. Gronvall, 'The Re-emergent H1N1 strain', https://jhu.pure.elsevier.com/en/publications/the-reemergent-1977-h1n1-strain-and-the-gain-of-function-debate.

25 Interview with Rick Ostveld, 2021.

26 If Not Us Then Who?, 'The Coalition to Prevent Pandemics at the Source calls on the United States Congress to Prioritize Pandemic Prevention', https://ifnotusthenwho.me, accessed 20 October 2022.

27 Interview with Walter Plowright, 2020.

CHAPTER 15

1 Mark Pallen, *The Last Days of Smallpox: Tragedy in Birmingham*, self-published, 2018, pp. 154–5.

2 Lynn C. Klotz, 'The pandemic risk of an accidental lab leak of enhanced flu virus: unacceptably high', https://thebulletin.org, 26 June 2020.

3 Alison Young, 'Newly disclosed CDC biolab failures "like a screenplay for a disaster movie"', https://eu.usatoday.com, 2 June 2016.

4 Alison Young and Jessica Blake, 'Near Misses at High Security Lab Illustrate Risk of Accidents With Coronaviruses', www.propublica. org, 17 August 2020.

5 Interview with Lynn C. Klotz, 2022.

6 Lynn C. Klotz and Edward J. Sylvester, 'The unacceptable risks of a man-made pandemic', https://thebulletin.org, 7 August 2012.

7 David Manheim and Gregory Lewis, 'High-risk human-caused pathogen exposure events 1976–2016', https://f1000research.com, 2021.

8 Interview with Philippa Lentzos, 2020.

9 R. M. Pike, 'Past and present hazards of working with infectious agents', *Archives of Pathology and Laboratory Medicine*, 102/7 (1978), https://pubmed.ncbi.nlm.nih.gov.

10 'Potential Laboratory-acquired Salmonella Infection at CDC', https://search.cdc.gov, 31 March 2016.

11 'What to know about arboviruses', www.medicalnewstoday.com, accessed 20 October 2022.

12 Karen B. Byers, 'Laboratory Acquired Infections 1979–2020', 60th Annual Biological Safety Conference, Albuquerque, 13–18 October 2017, https://absaconference.org.

13 'UN health agency: Hungarian scientist sickened by Ebola', https:// uk.news.yahoo.com, 20 April 2018.

14 Richard D. Henkel et al., 'Monitoring Select Agent Theft, Loss and Release Reports in the United States: 2004–2010', *Applied Biosafety*,

17/4 (2012), https://journals.sagepub.com; Byers, 'Laboratory Acquired Infections'.

15 Alison Young, 'Inside America's Secretive Biolabs', https://eu.usatoday.com, 11 July 2014.

16 Hoai-Tran Bui, 'CDC increases regulations after anthrax, smallpox scares', https://eu.usatoday.com, 11 July 2014.

17 Jocelyn Kaiser, 'Six vials of smallpox discovered in US Lab', www.sciencemag.org, 8 July 2014.

18 David Malakoff, 'CDC says 75 workers may have been exposed to anthrax', www.sciencemag.org, 17 June 2014.

19 Jim Miklaszewski and Maggie Fox, 'Live Anthrax Mistakenly Sent to US Labs', www.nbcnews.com, 27 May 2015.

20 Ian Sample, '100 safety breaches at UK labs handling deadly diseases', www.theguardian.com, 4 December 2014.

21 UK Government Review, 'Foot and Mouth Disease 2007: A Review and Lessons Learned', www.gov.uk, 2007.

22 Joel Wertheim, 'The re-emergence of H1N1 Influenza Virus in 1977: a cautionary tale for estimating divergence times using biologically unrealistic sampling dates', *PlosOne*, 17/5 (June 2010), https://journals.plos.org.

23 Michelle Rozo and Gigi Kwik Gronvall, 'The Reemergent 1977 H1N1 Strain and the Gain-of-Function Debate', https://www.ncbi.nlm.nih.gov/pmc/articles/PMC4542197/.

24 Ibid.

25 Anthony S. Fauci, Gary J. Nabel and Francis S. Collins, 'A flu virus risk worth taking', www.washingtonpost.com, 31 December 2011.

26 Paul Duprex et al., 'Gain-of-function experiments: time for a real debate', *Nat. Rev. Microbiol*, 13/1 (2015), https://pubmed.ncbi.nlm.nih.gov.

27 Cambridge Working Group, 'Statement on Creation of Potential Pandemic Pathogens 2014', www.cambridgeworkinggroup.org.

28 Ibid.

29 Kelsey Piper, 'Why Work Should Stop on Making Viruses', www.vox.com, 5 January 2020.

30 Ronnie Cummins and Alexis Baden-Mayer, 'COVID-19: Reckless "Gain-of-Function" Experiments Lie at the Root of the Pandemic', www.organicconsumers.org, 23 July 2020.

31 Laura H. Kahn, 'Creating dangerous viruses in the lab is a bad way to guard against future pandemics', https://thebulletin.org, 19 November 2021.

32 Ken Alibek, with Stephen Handelman, *Biohazard*, Arrow Books, London, 2000, pp. 70–86.

33 Jonathan B. Tucker, 'Biological weapons in the former Soviet Union: an interview with Dr. Kenneth Alibek', 1989, transcript at www.nonproliferation.org.

34 Li Xu, 'Analysis of Six Patients with Severe Pneumonia Caused by Unknown Viruses'. School of Clinical Medicine, Kunming Medical University, 2013, www.documentcloud.org.

35 WHO, 'WHO-convened Global Study of Origins of SARS-CoV-2: China Part', www.who.int, 14 January–10 February 2021.

36 Jonathan Latham and Alison Wilson, 'The case is building that Covid-19 had a lab origin', www.independentsciencenews.org, 2 June 2020.

37 Kai Kupferschmidt, 'How Canadian researchers reconstituted an extinct poxvirus for $100,000 using mail-order DNA', www.sciencemag.org, 6 July 2017.

38 Maggie Fox, 'Vials labeled "smallpox" found at vaccine research facility in Pennsylvania, CDC says', https://edition.cnn.com, 16 November 2021.

CHAPTER 16

1 Elizabeth Pennisi, 'A tropical parasitic disease has invaded Europe, thanks to a hybrid of two infectious worms', www.science.org, 28 August 2018.

2 Jérôme Boissier et al., 'Outbreak of urogenital schistosomiasis in Corsica (France): an epidemiological case study', *The Lancet*, 16/8 (August 2016), www.thelancet.com.

3 Nate Seltennch, 'Down to Earth: The Emerging Field of Planetary Health'. *Environmental Health Perspectives*, 126/7 (July 2018), www.ncbi.nlm.nih.gov.

4 Interview with Robert Horton, 2021.

5 Stephen Morse et al., 'Prediction and prevention of the next pandemic zoonosis', *The Lancet*, 380/9857 (December 2012), www.thelancet.com.

6 Astrid Wester, 'Antimicrobial Resistance in a One Health Perspective', from *International Encyclopaedia of Public Health* (2017), www.sciencedirect.com.

7 Laura H. Kahn, 'Confronting Zoonoses, Linking Human and Veterinary Medicine', *Emerging International Diseases*, 12/4 (April 2006), wwwnc.cdc.gov.

8 Interview with Dennis Carroll, 2021.

9 Ibid.

10 Kevin Berger, 'The Man Who Saw the Pandemic Coming', https://nautil.us, 13 March 2020.

11 Olga Jonas and Richard Seifman, 'Do we need a Global Virome Project?', *The Lancet*, 7/10 (October 2019).

12 Interview with Dennis Carroll, 2022.

13 Ibid.

14 Ibid.

15 Interview with Rick Bright, 2021.

16 Interview with Thomas Gillespie, 2022.

17 Ibid.

18 David W. Redding et al., 'Impacts of environmental and socio-economic factors on emergence and epidemic potential of Ebola in Africa', www.nature.com, 15 October 2019.

19 Interview with David Redding, 2021.

20 Interview with Kate Jones, 2021.

21 CDC, 'Selecting Viruses for the Seasonal Influenza Vaccine', www.cdc.gov, accessed 20 October 2022.

22 WHO, 'Water, Sanitation, and Hygiene in Health Care Facilities Practical Steps to Achieve Universal Access to Quality Care', https://apps.who.int, 2019.

23 Interview with Helen Clark, 2020.

24 Ibid.

25 Interview with Jonathan Quick, 2020.

26 Interview with Aaron Bernstein, 2022. See also science.org/doi/10.1126/scidv.abl4183.

27 Frieden, 'We share a Common Enemy'. Global health 2020.https://www.thinkglobalhealth.org/article/dr-tom-frieden-politics-epidemics 2020

28 Ibid.

CHAPTER 17

1 Stefan Dege, 'A place with no coronavirus restrictions', www.dw.com, 24 April 2020.

2 Alison Bray, 'Explosion of visitors hiking forests since pandemic – Coillte', www.independent.ie, 16 February 2021.

3 Catherine Arnold, 'In Pandemic, People Are Turning to Nature – Especially Women', www.uvm.edu, 16 December 2020.

4 UK Office of National Statistics. 'Lockdown Changed Our Relationship with Nature', www.ons.gov.uk, 26 April 2021.

5 Y. Otsuka et al., 'Shinrin-yoku (forest-air bathing and walking) effectively decreases blood glucose levels in diabetic patients', *International Journal of Biometeorology*, 41 (1998), https://link.springer.com.

6 J. Maas et al., 'Morbidity is related to a green living environment', *Journal of Epidemiology and Community Health*, 63/12 (2009), https://jech.bmj.com.

7 Andrea Faber Taylor and Francis Kuo, 'Children with Attention Disorders Concentrate Better After Walk in the Park', *Journal of Attention Disorders*, 12/5 (2009), https://journals.sagepub.com.

8 Yoko Tsunetsugu et al., 'Trends in research related to "Shinrin-yoku" (taking in the forest atmosphere or forest bathing) in Japan', *Environmental Health and Preventative Medicine*, 15/1 (January 2010), www.ncbi.nlm.nih.gov.

9 Jeffrey Craig et al., 'Natural environments, nature relatedness and the ecological theater: connecting satellites and sequencing to shinrin-yoku', *Journal of Physiological Anthropology*, 35/1 (2016), https://jphysiolanthropol.biomedcentral.com.

10 Joan Maloof, 'Perspectives: Take a Deep Breath', www.newscientist.com, 31 August 2005.

11 R. Aerts et al., 'Biodiversity and human health', *British Medical Bulletin*, 127 (1), 5–22. doi: 10.1093/bmb/ld.

12 Miyazaki Yoshifum, 'Japan for Sustainability 2011'. https://www.japanfs.org/en/news/archives/news_id030816.html.

13 Graham Rook, 'Old Friends Hypothesis', www.grahamrook.net, accessed 20 October 2022.

14 David Miller et al., 'Contribution of Green and Open Space to Public Health and Wellbeing: Final Report' (February 2014), www.hutton.ac.uk.

15 Marja Roslund et al., 'Biodiversity intervention enhances immune regulation and health-associated commensal microbiota among daycare children', *Science Advances*, 6/42 (14 October 2020), www. science.org.

16 Ibid.

17 L. Ruokolainen et al., 'Significant disparities in allergy prevalence and microbiota between the young people in Finnish and Russian Karelia', *Clinical and Experimental Allergy*, 47/5 (May 2017), https:// onlinelibrary.wiley.com.

18 Rachel Shabi, 'Sanctuary in the city: how urban parks saved our summer', www.theguardian.com, 9 August 2020.

19 UK Government Official Statistics, 'Monitor of Engagement with the Natural Environment pilot study: visits to the natural environment by children', www.gov.uk. 10 February 2016.

20 Qian Gao et al., 'Changes in Time Spent Outdoors During the Daytime in Rural Populations in Four Geographically Distinct Regions in China: A Retrospective Study', *Photochemistry and Photobiology*, 93/2 (March/April 2017), https://onlinelibrary.wiley. com.

21 Peter Kahn, *Technological Nature; Adaptation and the Future of Human Life*, MIT Press, Cambridge, MA, 2011.

22 Ibid.

23 WHO, 'Urban green spaces and health: a review of evidence' (2016), www.euro.who.int.

24 Catharine Ward Thompson, 'Linking landscape and health: the recurring theme', *Landscape and Urban Planning*, 99 (2011), http:// blogs.ubc.ca.

25 Ibid.

26 Ibid.

27 Ibid.

CHAPTER 18

1 Interview with Sabarmatee Apa, 2019.

2 UN Environment Programme. 'Land Degradation' factsheet, https:// wedocs.unep.org, accessed 20 October 2022.

3 Simon Ferrier, 'Prioritising Where to Restore Earth's Ecosystems', www.nature.com, 14 October 2020.

4 Tim Christofferson in Patrick Greenfield, 'World must rewild on massive scale to heal nature and climate, says UN', *Guardian*, 3 June 2021, https://www.theguardian.com/environment/2021/jun/03/rewild-on-massive-scale-to-heal-nature-and-climate-says-un-decade-on-ecosystem-restoration-aoe.

5 Annelies Sewell et al., 'Goals and Commitments for the Restoration Decade', www.pbl.nl, October 2020.

6 World Economic Forum, 'China Has Sent 60,000 Soldiers to Plant Trees', www.weforum.org, 16 February 2018.

7 UN Convention to Combat Desertification, 'The Great Green Wall', www.greatgreenwall.org, accessed 20 October 2022.

8 Chris Reij et al., 'Agroenvironmental Transformation in the Sahel', https://core.ac.uk, 2020.

9 Interview with Wangari Maathai, 2011.

10 Ibid.

11 Ibid.

12 Ibid.

13 Ibid.

14 Ibid.

15 Chris Llang, 'Greenpeace rejects the one trillion trees campaign: "Treewashing the climate crisis with promises of large tree plantations"', https://redd-monitor.org, 20 March 2020.

16 Graham Lawson, 'Rescue plan for nature: How to fix the biodiversity crisis', www.newscientist.com, 17 February 2021.

17 'Grasslands: An emerging frontier for nature-based Carbon Credits', https://carboncredits.com, 30 December 2021.

18 Amnesty International, 'Case Studies: Palm Oil and Human Rights Abuses', www.amnesty.org, 30 November 2016.

19 Guy Shrubsole, 'Finding the Land to Double Tree Cover', https://policy.friendsoftheearth.uk, 17 March 2020.

20 Interview with Graham Knight, 2016.

21 Interview with John Everitt, 2016.

22 Ibid.

23 Interview with Chris Reij, 2014.

24 Interview with Chris Reij, 2021.

25 Interview with Alfredo Cunhal, 2020.

26 www.globalhungerindex.org/case-studies/2018-malawi.html.

27 Ibid.

28 Tilele Stevens and Madani Kaveh. 'Future climate impacts on maize farming and food security in Malawi', *Scientific Reports*, 6 (8 November 2016), www.nature.com.

29 Interview Stacia and Kristof Nordin, 2019.

30 Interview with Luwayo Biswick, 2021.

CONCLUSION

1 Mark Woolhouse et al., 'Human viruses: discovery and emergence', *Philos. Trans. R. Soc. Lond. B. Biol. Sci.*, 367/1904 (October 2012), www.ncbi.nlm.nih.gov.

2 Colin Carlson et al., 'The future of zoonotic risk prediction', *Philos. Trans. R. Soc. Lond. B. Biol. Sci.*, 376/1837 (November 2021), https://royalsocietypublishing.org.

3 William Sutherland et al., 'Identification of 100 fundamental ecological questions', *Journal of Ecology*, 101/1 (January 2013), https://besjournals.onlinelibrary.wiley.com.

4 Piero Scaruffi, 'Wars and Casualties of the 20th and 21st Centuries', www.scaruffi.com, 2009.

5 Harry Kretchmer, '5 urgent actions to stop future pandemics crushing the global economy', www.weforum.org, 12 October 2020.

6 Heeso Joo et al., 'Economic Impact of the 2015 MERS Outbreak on the Republic of Korea's Tourism-Related Industries', *Health Security*, 17/2 (April 2019), www.researchgate.net.

7 Mehmood Ul-Hassan Khan, 'Economic Cost of Bird Flu', www.mediamonitors.net, 13 February 2004.

8 'U.S. Military Spending/Defense Budget 1960–2022', www.macrotrends.ne, accessed 20 October 2022; Peter Sands et al., 'Assessment of economic vulnerability to infectious disease crises', *The Lancet*, 388/10058 (2016), www.thelancet.com.

9 Dimitrios Gouglas et al., 'Estimating the cost of vaccine development against epidemic infectious diseases: a cost minimisation study', *The Lancet*, 6/12 E1386–E1396 (1 December 2018), www.thelancet.com.

10 Colin Carlson et al., 'Climate change will drive novel cross-species viral transmission'. www.biorxiv.org, 19 April 2021.

BIBLIOGRAPHY

Alibek, Ken, *Biohazard*, Arrow Books, London, 2000

Barnes, Ethne, *Diseases and Human Evolution*, University of New Mexico, Albuquerque, 2007

Bartlett, Sheridan, and David Satterthwaite, *Cities on a Finite Planet*, Earthscan, London, 2016

Baskin, Yvonne, *A Plague of Rats and Rubbervines*, Island Press, Washington, DC, 2002

Bate, Jonathan, *The Song of the Earth*, Picador, London, 2000

Blanc, Guillaume, *The Invention of Green Colonialism*, Polity, Cambridge, 2016

Boulter, Michael, *Extinction*, Fourth Estate, London, 2002

Bright, Chris, *Life Out of Bounds*, Worldwatch, London, 1998

Burger, William, *Complexity in Biodiversity*, Prometheus, London, 2016

Challenger, Melanie, *On Extinction*, Granta, London, 2011

Christakis, Nicholas, *Apollo's Arrow*, Little, Brown, New York, 2020

Clark, J. F. M., *Bugs and the Victorians*, Yale University Press, New Haven, 2009

Cook, Noble David, *Born to Die: Disease and New World Conquest*, Cambridge University Press, Cambridge, 1998

Cowden, James, and John Duffy, *The Elder Dempster Fleet History, 1852–1985*, Mallett & Bell, Norfolk, 1986

Crawford, Dorothy, *Deadly Companions*, Oxford University Press, Oxford, 2007

Cregan-Reid, Vybarr, *Primate Change*, Cassell, London, 2018

Crosby, Alfred, *Ecological Imperialism*, Cambridge University Press, Cambridge, 1986

Dartnell, Lewis, *Origins*, Vintage, London, 2019

Davies, Hunter, *In Search of Columbus*, Sinclair-Stevenson, London, 1992

Davis, Wade, *One River*, Vintage, London, 2014

Deville, Patrick, *Plague and Cholera*, Little, Brown, New York 2014

Diamond, Jared, *Guns, Germs, and Steel*, Vintage, London, 1998

Farmer, Paul, *Fevers, Feuds and Diamonds*, F&G, London, 2020

Farrar, Jeremy, *Spike*, Profile, London, 2021

France, David, *How to Survive a Plague*, Picador, London, 2016

Garrett, Laurie, *The Coming Plague*, Picador, London, 1994

Geall, Sam, *China and the Environment*, Zed Books, London, 2013

Goldsmith, Edward, *The Way*, Rider, London, 1992

Gott, Richard, *Cuba*, Yale University Press, New Haven, 2005

Greger, Michael, *How to Survive a Panic*, Flatiron, New York, 2020

Grifo, Francesca, and Joshua Rosenthal, *Biodiversity and Human Health*, Island Press, Washington, DC, 1997

Haley, Bruce, *The Healthy Body and Victorian Culture*, Harvard University Press, Cambridge, MA, 1979

Hanley, Paul, *Man of the Trees*, University of Regina Press, Regina, 2018

Harper, Kyle, *The Fate of Rome*, Princeton University Press, Princeton, 2017

Hillel, Daniel, *Out of the Earth*, Aurum, London, 1992

Honigsbaum, Mark, *The Fever Trail*, F&G, London, 2001

Honigsbaum, Mark, *The Pandemic Century*, Penguin, Harmondsworth, 2019

Hooper, Edward, *The River*, Little, Brown, New York, 2000

Horton, Richard, *The Covid-19 Catastrophe*, Polity, Cambridge, 2021

Hume, Julian, and Michael Waters, *Extinct Birds*, Poyser, London, 2012

James, Lawrence, *Empires of the Sun*, Weidenfeld & Nicolson, London, 2016

Johnson, James, *The Influence of Tropical Climates on European Constitutions*, Collins & Co., New York, 1826

Kennedy, Roger, *Mr Jefferson's Lost Cause*, Oxford University Press, Oxford, 2004

Kopenawa, Davi, and Bruce Albert, *The Falling Sky*, Harvard University Press, Cambridge, MA, 2010

Kucharski, Adam, *The Rules of Contagion*, Wellcome, London, 2020

Lee, Jon D., *Epidemic An Epidemic of Rumors*, Utah State University Press, Logan, Utah, 2012

Leick, Gwendolyn, *Mesopotamia: The Invention of the City*, Penguin, Harmondsworth, 2002

Lever, Christopher, *They Dined on Eland*, Quiller, London, 1992

Levy, Elinor, and Mark Fischetti, *The New Killer Diseases*, Three Rivers Press, New York, 2004

Linden, Eugene, *Fire and Flood*, Allen Lane, London, 2020

Little, Charles E., *The Dying of the Trees*, Viking, London, 1995

Lymbery, Philip, and Isabel Oakeshott, *Farmageddon*, Bloomsbury, London, 2014

Lymbery, Philip, *Dead Zone*, Bloomsbury, London, 2017

Maathai, Wangari, *Unbowed*, Heinemann, London, 2007

MacIntosh, Donald, *Travels in the White Man's Grave*, Wilson, London, 1999

Magner, Lois, *A History of Medicine*, Dekker, New York, 1992

Mazza, Giuseppe, and Elena Tricario, *Invasive Species and Human Health*, Cabi CABI, Wallingford, 2021

McCormick, Joseph B., and Susan Fisher-Hoch, *Level 4 Virus-Hunters of the CDC*, Barnes &, Noble, New York, 1999

McLean, George, and Ronald Garrett, *Plant Virus Epidemics*, Academic Press, San Diego, 1996

McNeill, Donald G. Jr, *Zika*, Norton, London, 2016

McNeill, William, *Plagues and Peoples*, Peregrine, London, 1976

Mercola, Joseph, and Ronnie Cummings, *The Truth About Covid-19*, Chelsea Green Publishing, White River Junction, 2021

Middleton, Nick, *Extremes Along the Silk Road*, John Murray, London, 2005

Mithen, Steven, *After the Ice*, Harvard University Press, Cambridge, MA, 2006

Montgomery, David R., and Anne Bikle, *The Hidden Half of Nature*, Norton, London, 2016

Muir-Woord, Robert, *The Cure for Catastrophe*, Simon & Schuster, New York, 2018

Myers, Samuel, and Howard Frumkin, *Planetary Health*, Island Press, Washington, DC, 2021

Novotny, Vojtech, *Notebooks from New Guinea*, Oxford University Press, Oxford, 2009

Olmsted, Fred, *Walks and Talks of an American Farmer in England*, 1852, Forgotten Books, London

Orent, Wendy, *Plague*, Free Press, New York, 2005

Orion, Tao, *Beyond the War on Invasive Species*, Chelsea Green Publishing, White River Junction, Vermont, 2015

Osborn, Ann, *The Four Seasons of the U'wa*, Sean Kingston Publishing, Canon Pyon, Herefordshire, 2009

Osterholm, Michael, *Deadliest Enemy*, John Murray, London, 2017

Parker, Matthew, *The Sugar Barons*, Hutchinson, London, 2011

Pearce, Fred, *Deep Jungle*, Eden Project, Cornwall, 2006

Pearce, Fred, *The Landgrabbers*, Eden Project, Cornwall, 2012

Pearce, Fred, *The New Wild*, Icon, London, 2015

Peters, C. J., *Virus Hunter*, Anchor, New York, 1997

Petersen, Dale, *Eating Apes*, University of California Press, Stanford, 2003

Piot, Peter, *No Time to Lose*, Norton, New York, 2012

Pollen, Mark, *The Last Days of Smallpox*, self-published, 2018

Porritt, Jonathan, *Hope in Hell*, Simon &, Schuster, New York, 2020

Preston, Richard, *Panic in Level 4*, Random House, London, 2009

Preston, Richard, *The Hot Zone*, Corgi, London, 1995

Pringle, Peter, *The Murder of Nikolai Vavilov*, Simon & Schuster, New York, 2008

Quammen, David, *Ebola*, Bodley Head, London, 2018

Quammen, David, *Spillover*, Vintage, London, 2013

Rackham, Oliver, *The Ash Tree*, Little Toller, Beaminster, Dorset, 2014

Ramen, William, *Justinian's Flea*, Jonathan Cape, London, 2007

Reader, John, *Cities*, Heinemann, London, 2004

Reichholf, Josef, *The Disappearance of Butterflies*, Polity, Cambridge, 2021

Reij, Chris, *Sustaining the Soil*, Earthscan, London, 1996

Richards, Paul, *Ebola*, Zed Books, London, 2016

Ryan, Frank, *Virusphere*, HarperCollins, London, 2019

Scott, Richard Shaw, *Planet of the Bugs*, University of Chicago Press, Chicago, 2014

Senthilingam, Meera, *Outbreaks and Epidemics*, Icon, London, 2020

Shuker, Karl, *The Lost Ark*, Collins, London, 1993

Simberloff, Daniel, *Invasive Species*, Oxford University Press, Oxford, 2013

Spinney, Laura, *Pale Rider*, Vintage, London, 2017

Stolzenburg, William, *Rat Island*, Bloomsbury, London, 2011

Stone, Roger, and Claudia d'Andrea, *Tropical Forests and the Human Spirit*, University of California Press, Stanford, 2002

Sykes, Rebecca, *Kindred*, Bloomsbury, London, 2020

Thomas, William, *Man's Role in Changing the Face of the Earth*, Vol. 1, University of Chicago Press, Chicago, 1972

Tomkins, Peter, and Christopher Bird, *Secrets of the Soil*, Viking, London, 1989

Trefon, Theodore, *Congo's Environmental Paradox*, Zed Books, London, 2016

Tudge, Colin, *The Great Re-think*, Pari Publishing, Pari, Tuscany, 2021

Turner, Judy, *Animals, Ethics and Trade*, Earthscan, London, 2006

Vince, Gaia, *Adventures in the Anthropocene*, Chatto & Windus, London, 2014

Wallace, Rob, *Big Farms Make Big Flu*, Monthly Review Press, New York, 2021

Wallace, Rob, *Dead Epidemiologists*, Monthly Review Press, New York, 2020

Watson, Peter, *The Great Divide*, Weidenfeld & Nicolson, New York, 2012

Watts, Jonathan, *When a Billion Chinese Jump*, Faber & Faber, London 2010

Wilson, Edward O., *Anthill*, Norton, London, 2010

Wilson, Edward O., *The Future of Life*, Little, Brown, New York, 2002

Wolfe, Nathan, *The Viral Storm*, Allen Lane, London, 2011

INDEX

A NOTE ON THE TYPE

The text of this book is set Adobe Garamond. It is one of several versions of Garamond based on the designs of Claude Garamond. It is thought that Garamond based his font on Bembo, cut in 1495 by Francesco Griffo in collaboration with the Italian printer Aldus Manutius. Garamond types were first used in books printed in Paris around 1532. Many of the present-day versions of this type are based on the *Typi Academiae* of Jean Jannon cut in Sedan in 1615.

Claude Garamond was born in Paris in 1480. He learned how to cut type from his father and by the age of fifteen he was able to fashion steel punches the size of a pica with great precision. At the age of sixty he was commissioned by King Francis I to design a Greek alphabet, and for this he was given the honourable title of royal type founder. He died in 1561.